Y0-BRR-555

THE PRACTICE
OF
AROMATHERAPY

THE PRACTICE
OF
AROMATHERAPY

Holistic Health and the Essential Oils of
Flowers and Herbs

Jean Valnet, M.D.

Translated from the French by
Robin Campbell and Libby Houston

Edited by Robert Tisserand

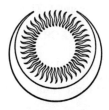

Destiny Books
New York

Destiny Books
377 Park Avenue South
New York, New York 10016

Originally published in France under the title *Aromathérapie*
by Librairie Maloine, S.A.
Copyright © 1980 Dr. Jean Valnet
English Translation Copyright © 1982 The C.W. Daniel Company Ltd.

All rights reserved. No part of this book may be reproduced or utilized in
any form or by any means, electronic or mechanical, including photo-
copying and recording, or by any information storage and retrieval
system, without permission in writing from the publisher. Inquiries should
be addressed to Destiny Books.

Library of Congress Cataloging in Publication Data
Valnet, Jean
   The practice of aromatherapy.

   Translation of: Aromathérapie.
   Bibliography: p.
   Includes index.
   1. Essences and essential oils—Therapeutic use.
2. Aromatic plants—Therapeutic use. I. Title.
RM666.A68V3413   615'.321   82-4968
ISBN 0-89281-026-2   AACR2

10 9 8 7 6 5 4 3 2

Printed in the United States of America
Destiny Books is a division of Inner Traditions International Ltd.

CONTENTS

CONTENTS

FOREWORD

Les médecins pourraient tirer des odeurs
plus d'usages qu'ils ne font

Montaigne

Forgotten and ignored for many years, aromatic essences are coming back into their own, for many researchers and for a large section of public opinion, as the stars of medicine. Faced with a mounting toll of complications known to have been caused by aggressively synthesised chemical medications, many patients are now unwilling to be treated except by natural therapies, foremost among which plants and their essences have a rightful place.

It is worth reflecting on the mixed fates of the many types of medicine and medicament human beings have developed for their fellows since the world began. Again and again we find ourselves brought back to the medicine of ordinary simple folk, if indeed we have ever completely abandoned it – that medicine which Henri Leclerc has described as "so dear to our ancestors and, in the light of current methods, stripped of its legends and obscurities". Most often we return to it as a last resort, when some serious condition has failed to respond to the whole gamut of modern therapies. We should obviously do better and waste less time if, for a number of diseases, we made it our starting-point.

This book, I trust, will in certain of its aspects serve as one of those direct links between modern knowledge and the experience of the past. Recent discoveries, such as those which have shown the existence of hormones and antibiotic principles in many plants and essences, suggest that we should have been wary of making snap judgements about how such medicines work. We have now been given a simple and logical account of their action, through various hormonal correspondences, on both the physical body and the psyche. Numerous experiments enable us to explain some of the age-old treatments which until now were dismissed with a smile – the sachets of garlic or other plants, for instance, which our forefathers used to hang round the necks of children with worms or used more generally during epidemics. We shall see how it is possible to explain, in cases of gout, certain aches and pains, inability to urinate, the curative action of the various traditional poultices whose only constituents were boiled crushed herbs.

Similarly, in a different territory, gallstone-sufferers have claimed that under the hands of magnetic healers they have felt their stones disintegrate and their discomfort vanish. Who has not heard such stories and laughed outright at them? Well, "experiments are being carried out in a surgical clinic in Budapest on the analysis of gallstones by ultrasonics. Calculi extracted by surgery have already been exposed to ultrasonic waves under artificial conditions corresponding to those of the gall-bladder. Among the calculi – which are of three types – those of the first, and commonest, category (cholesterol-pigment-calcareous) were *reduced to powder after 2–5 exposures to ultrasonic waves*; those of the other two categories were found to have crumbled." *(Presse Médicale,* 1962).

"Gentle reader," I would say after Montaigne, "this is an honest book." In 1957 when I was serving as doctor, rank of major, in the French Army Ministry, a colonel's wife whom I knew to have spent months in vain consulting various skin specialists about the persistent eczema on her forearms came in one morning to dumbfound me. She had just returned from visiting a village near Bearn and called to show me her arms, innocent of any mark, the skin restored to health.

Before I could speak, she launched into the explanation:

"Doctor, I know you never laugh at the outlandish treatments people think worth a try. . . . Remember my eczema? Look at it now!"

The skin I saw before me was very fair and agreeably tinted. In my mind's eye I could still see the repellent reddish lesions with their scattering of bright yellow scabs.

"This is what happened – and please forgive me for being unfaithful to you. . . . Somebody once told me about an old fellow in a little village quite a long way from here with a reputation for curing eczema, so I went to see him. Now don't laugh: he lifted me up on his back, carried me like that right round his garden and brought me back into his house."

I was somewhat surprised, but let her continue.

" 'There you are, ma'am, that's all,' he said. 'Tomorrow or the day after it'll all be gone.' That was three days ago – and now, you see?"

What can I say?

The aim of this book is not to offer explanations for such phenomena which completely baffle us, and which will, no doubt, remain for a long time to come as far beyond the scope of the general practitioner as the art of a Gad, a Gus or a Pouzet – as surely as the magnetism of a Clemenceau or a Napoleon eludes the grasp of ordinary men.

And yet the informed use of plants and essences can produce effects which to the layman appear just as "miraculous". The Ancient Egyptians already knew how to anaesthetise with full-bodied maceration of plants.

In his many books, Professor Léon Binet, a former Dean of the Faculty of Medicine in Paris, has commented time and again on the extraordinary healing properties of the substances found in plants.

The names of the most eminent researchers, doctors, biologists and pharmacists, continually appear among the authors of the numerous works that deal with plants and essential oils.

I would not attempt to mention them all here, nor restrict the list to France. We shall come across many others along the way, but Chamberland, Cadéac and Meunier, Courmont, Morel, Rochaix and Bay, Cazin, Binet, Balansard, Caujolle, Chabrol and Dorvault are the names which anyone making a serious study of plants and their constituents will find continually recurring; likewise those of Goris, Duquesnois, Perrot, Meurisse, Lemaire, Lian, Loeper, H. Leclerc, Fournier, R. M. Gattefossé, F. Decaux, R. Paris[1], Quevauvillers, Guyon, Carraz, Valette, R. Moreau and a number of others who have contributed to the present state of knowledge in this field.

Many researchers, many of them in the universities, have made plants their subject and published their studies. Among them I should mention J. Berbaud, Bézanger-Beauquesne, Debelmas, P. Delaveau, B. Drevon, R. B. Henry, A. Foucaud, J. Kerharo, J. M. Pelt, A. de Sambucy, H. Pourrat. . .

The names of Gatti and Cajola, Carosi, Remigio Banal, Novi and Paolo Rovesti will be known in Italy; those of Kobert, Bruning and Arno Müller in Germany, and in America and Great Britain those of Martindale, Miller, Read, Rideal, Tanner and Willey. All these have written numerous works and articles concerning the study of plant essences.

At Toulouse, Professor Caujolle has for many years presided as chairman of the board examining theses devoted to the study of vegetable essences, including those of Ms Porcher-Pimpart, R. Cazel, A. Azaloux and Cathala. At Rennes, Professor Grégoire sponsored Sarbach's thesis on the antiseptic and bactericidal action of 54 essential oils. At Montpellier, a truly neo-Hippocratic school has been set up with Professors Guerrier and Pagés among others at its head, and has published the results of its work.

In Dakar, J. Kerharo, Professor of Pharmacology, has spent years in patient research. Following many articles and *Aromatherapy and Gem Therapy in the traditional Pharmacopoeia of Senegal* which appeared in the journal of tropical agriculture and practical botany in 1971, he published with J. G. Adam in 1974 a monumental work: *The Traditional Pharmacopoeia of Senegal* (publ. Vigot).

The school at Lyons for its part, as inheritor of the traditions of R. M. Gattefossé – to whom we owe the term *Aromatherapy* itself – carries on the work of its predecessor.

In other countries the picture is similar: the Italian school, for

1 Professor René Paris, whose name cannot be ignored by anyone writing about plants, is holder of the chair of *Materia Medica* in the Faculty of Pharmacy in paris. We owe to him the only World Museum of Phytotherapy, consulted in their hundreds by doctors and pharmacists from France and abroad as well as students. (4 Av. de l'Observatoire – 75005 Paris).

instance, with Professors Rovesti of Milan, Cerevoli of Padua, Benedicenti and others.

In Belgium the movement has been much slower to take root, in spite of the efforts of Marc Danval, Georges Wielemans, Janine Modave, J. Kother, J. L. Lechat, M. Grodent, Ch. Van Hoof, A. Antoine, Ph. Genaert, N. P. Ketelbuters and F. Wangermée.

I could give further examples from Russia and the United States. . . . In short, we are witnessing a world-wide blossoming of a new Hippocratic approach, or, as Professor Savy has described it, "a collaboration with nature" in the work of healing. Without denying the value of physico-chemical knowledge obtained in the laboratory, we are making use of the weapons Nature offers us, no longer, this time, in an empirical manner but more rationally, on a scientific basis.

And so in the course of this book I shall be giving explanations, made possible by modern research, of numerous traditional treatments hither-to ignored or denied – in spite of the results they have always produced.

"There is nothing less scientific than to deny something because it can-not be explained." In spite of the truth of this saying, many more or less learned – or ignorant – people have laughed at undeniable results simply because we were still unable to give adequate explanations. "In a period of scientific discoveries as fruitful as our own," wrote Léon Binet, "it is often hard to avoid excessive pride and to remember, with Pascal, that 'the succession of men down the centuries may be considered as one single man who exists eternally and is in a continuous state of learning'." "If we are tempted to smile," said Henri Leclerc, "then we should do it discreetly, imagining the impression the medical terminology of which we are so proud will have on our great-grandchildren".

It was that reminder which led me to reject as far as I could the use of hermetic medical terms in this book. For those terms I have felt bound to use, I have included a glossary at the end.

For while I have certainly written this book for my colleagues, it has also been intended *above all* for the general public.

The well-spring, after all, rises from below, even in therapeutics. Often the patient's own opinion influences the kind of treatment he wishes to see administered. "The public are always the first to know, even if they are told nothing." wrote Mike Waltari (in *Sinhoué the Egyptian*).

Normal *preventive medicine*, which consists in giving healthy people drugs and injections of products *whose future effects are unpredictable*, is an aberration. Bringing about change by non-toxic means is the only efficacious course, among which aromatic plants and their essences have been, are, and will remain in the front rank.

If there are signs of a return to natural methods of treatment, it is still far from being universal. On a recent trip to Canada, I overheard a doctor giving a mother this advice: "If your children get a cold, give them these antibiotic tablets at once '. And the doctor brought from his bag a box without even a label on it!

*   *   *   *

Essences are usually obtained by distillation of the plants and, in the case of most of the plants considered in this book, are generally prescribed in the form of drops, *perles* or capsules. Perhaps it will seem strange that I have devoted separate sections to garlic, onion and camomile when these are practically never prescribed by doctors.

It is because the action of these plants and seasonings too is partly due to their aromatic *essences.*

Very often an effective method of treatment involves no more than the daily use in the kitchen of garlic, cloves, sage, rosemary, thyme, savory and many other herbs or seasonings, and this is why in the chapter dealing with the specific essences I have allowed some space to other ways of using the plants which produce them. Apart from infusions, decoctions and powders, fumigations, liniments and baths achieve their effects by means of the volatile oils they release.

I must at this stage make it clear that this book in no way claims to replace the difficult art of the therapist. "All is poison, nothing is poison," said Paracelsus, and in reality the dosage is all-important. For natural essences,if used carelessly, are just as likely to be toxic. Workers engaged in handling and packing vanilla beans, for instance, are subject to various sudden illnesses which may be classed under the heading of "vanillin", consisting of severe headaches, gastro-intestinal disorders and total though temporary loss of eyebrows. An overdose of saffron can produce cerebral excitation liable to trigger off convulsions, delirium and even death. Cadéac and Meunier have demonstrated that marjoram essence, which is antispasmodic, can in high doses become stupefacient. Even in weak doses the essences of sage, rosemary and hyssop can produce a tendency to epilepsy under certain conditions and in persons whose resistance is low.

Following the same line of thought, I should not pass over a curious incident from my own experience. In July 1959, on the occasion of the great annual fête at the Military School of la Flèche, a woman came to consult me about a severe case of nettlerash which had suddenly appeared on her forearms. I could not pinpoint the origin of her allergy. Neither diet, nor lipstick, nailvarnish, nor perfume – nothing could set me on the right track.

The same phenomenon was to recur a few years later, and this set me thinking.

Having gathered all the data I could, I found the cause to be a hypersensitivity to lime-blossom. Three times in eleven years this woman had happened to linger under a flowering lime-tree.

That said, in spite of the rare problems encountered in the use of plants and essences, "doctors and chemists will be surprised at the wide range of odoriferous substances which may be used medicinally," wrote R. M. Gattefossé, "and at the great variety of their chemical functions. Besides the antiseptic and antimicrobial properties of which use is currently made, the essential oils are also antitoxic and antiviral; they have a powerful energising effect and possess an undeniable cicatrising property. In the future their role will be even greater."

Montaigne was saying much the same thing when he wrote "doctors could make much greater use of odours than they do, for I have often noticed that they alter my state of being and act upon my spirits according to their variety."

Obviously Montaigne was ignorant of the modern research which has explained the action of plant essences on mind and body by the discovery of their hormonal and other principles. Present-day analysis has borne out his observations.

It has become commonplace to point out that traditional wisdom, in default of Science, continues to astound the impartial observer. How were our ancestors able to prescribe with such certainty and to such beneficial effect, knowing nothing of the chemical composition of the substances they administered? Experience was evidently considered sufficient explanation: when a child falls and hits his head you kiss the spot because you know it to have a calming effect.

But perhaps the Ancients knew more than we imagine and that knowledge has been lost or burned, for example, in the course of wars.

Besides, neither machines nor subtle analyses, counts nor diagrams can, curiously enough, altogether replace man in a number of everyday tasks.

Take chromatography, the method by which the different constituents of a liquid are distinguished in order to find out its composition and detect any falsities. The apparatus currently in use is extremely delicate and of the greatest possible precision; it has become as indispensable in research laboratories as it is to the services of the police (who, it seems, have only two at their disposal in the whole of France when private laboratories sometimes possess several!).

To continue, when the object is to analyse an aromatic essence intended for consumption (and I may say they generally carry the label "pure and natural" on the authority of the manufacturer when they are often adulterated), the chromatographic method is used to examine the succession of peaks obtained on a moving graph. You would expect it to be sufficient to compare the "curve" with the image type given by the truly pure and natural essence as reference.

But go along to one of these control laboratories one day, and you will observe that alongside the machine which is supposed to be infallible there is always a "nose" – i.e., a man or woman of highly specialised skills who for every individual graph will always sniff at the vapour which is given off. And it is the "nose" which says "the apparatus is right", or, if not, will correct the information given.

It is the same with every piece of machinery designed to take the place of men, some of which are even capable of rectifying their own mistakes. But when some readjustment is beyond their powers and they cannot resume their proper function, the technician still has to be brought in.

The technician is a human being who can follow many lines of thought, comparing and assessing in a way the machine can never do. All in all, there is still hope for the animal brain moulded as it is according to the most ancient laws.

Enough of that. I have before me now part of a book dating from the end of the last century. Compiled by a pharmacist – manufacturer of restoratives, sedatives, circulatory tonics – in fact, of numerous medicaments covering the whole range of pathology, the work is aimed primarily at promoting the author's own products to the exclusion of all others. As for impartiality and the scientific spirit, one would have to look elsewhere.

This pharmacist-salesman had obviously made a dedicated study of minerals, powdered bone and bromides, excellent therapeutic substances in their own right. But doubtless having no time to study the rest, he rejects them out of hand.

And so he warns his readers of the dangers of angelica, Chinese aniseed and basil, cabbage and capers, celery, chervil, cinnamon, cumin, fennel and ginger, lemons and onions, mulberries, parsnips, parsley, tarragon, tomatoes, thyme ... the entire list would cover pages.

And why? Because of the aromatic essences contained within these herbs, fruits and vegetables.

For this pseudo-authority but cunning shark, all plants containing essences are toxic. He certainly deserves a posthumous medal for services to the synthetic chemical industry for which he undoubtedly prepared the ground.

The sole objectives of this book, throughout its entire length, are to be useful and to remain scientific. I must stress particularly that I have no intention of stirring up controversy.

Moreover, it is in no way my purpose to advertise this or that product. If I have occasionally mentioned a few proprietary medicaments, it is to the sole end of assisting the reader newly fired with enthusiasm for the practice of aromatherapy on his way.

English and Botanical Names of Plants

ANISEED....................................	*Pimpinella anisum*
BASIL..	*Ocimum basilicum*
BERGAMOT	*Citrus bergamia*
BORNEO CAMPHOR, also Borneol....................................	Extract of *Dryobalanops camphora*
CAJUPUT..................................	*Melaleuca leucodendron*
CAMOMILE, ROMAN................	*Anthemis nobilis*
CAMOMILE, GERMAN	*Matricaria chamomilla*
CARAWAY	*Carum carvi*
CINNAMON OF CEYLON	*Cinnamomum zeylanicum*
CLOVE......................................	*Eugenia caryophyllata*
CORIANDER	*Coriandrum sativum*
CYPRESS...................................	*Cupressus sempervirens*
EUCALYPTUS............................	*Eucalyptus globulus*
FENNEL	*Foeniculum vulgare*
GARLIC....................................	*Allium sativum*
GERANIUM	*Pelargonium odorantissimum*
GINGER	*Zingiber officinale*
HYSSOP....................................	*Hyssopus officinalis*
JUNIPER	*Juniperus communis*
LAVENDER	*Lavandula officinalis*
LAVENDER-COTTON...............	*Santolina chamaecyparissus*
LEMON.....................................	*Citrus limonum*
LEMONGRASS	*Andropogon citratus, Cymbopogon citratus*
MARJORAM	*Origanum marjorana*
NIAOULI	*Melaleuca viridiflora*
NUTMEG	*Myristica fragrans*
ONION......................................	*Allium cepa*
ORANGE BLOSSOM	*Citrus aurantium, Citrus bigaradia*
ORIGANUM	*Origanum vulgare, (O. floribundum, O. glandulosum)*
PEPPERMINT	*Mentha piperita*
PINE...	*Pinus sylvestris*
ROSEMARY...............................	*Rosmarinus officinalis*
SAGE	*Salvia officinalis*
SANDALWOOD	*Santalum album, S. spicatum*
SAVORY, also Winter Savory	*Satureia montana*
TARRAGON..............................	*Artemisia dracunculus*
THUJA, also Arbor vitae..............	*Thuja occidentalis*
THYME......................................	*Thymus vulgaris*
TURPENTINE, or Terebinth.......	Resins of various species of *Pinus* and others
YLANG-YLANG	*Canangium odoratum*

Botanical and English Names of Plants and Essences

Allium cepa	ONION
Allium sativum	GARLIC
Andropogon citratus	LEMONGRASS
Anthemis nobilis	ROMAN CAMOMILE
Artemisia dracunculus	TARRAGON
Canangium odoratum	YLANG-YLANG
Carum carvi	CARAWAY
Cinnamomum zeylanicum	CINNAMON OF CEYLON
Citrus aurantium, C. bigaradia	ORANGE BLOSSOM
Citrus bergamia	BERGAMOT
Citrus limonum	LEMON
Coriandrum sativum	CORIANDER
Cupressus sempervirens	CYPRESS
Cymbopogon citratus	LEMONGRASS
Dryobalanops camphora	BORNEO CAMPHOR
Eucalyptus globulus	EUCALYPTUS
Eugenia caryophyllata	CLOVE
Foeniculum vulgare	FENNEL
Hyssopus officinalis	HYSSOP
Juniperus communis	JUNIPER
Lavandula officinalis	LAVENDER
Matricaria chamomilla	GERMAN CAMOMILE
Melaleuca leucodendron	CAJUPUT
Melaleuca viridiflora	NIAOULI
Mentha piperita	PEPPERMINT
Myristica fragrans	NUTMEG
Ocimum basilicum	BASIL
Origanum marjorana	MARJORAM
Origanum vulgare, (*O. floribundum O. glandulosum*)	ORIGANUM
Pelargonium odorantissimum	GERANIUM
Pimpinella anisum	ANISEED
Pinus sylvestris	PINE
Rosmarinus officinalis	ROSEMARY
Salvia officinalis	SAGE
Santalum album, S. spicatum	SANDALWOOD
Santolina chamaecyparissus	LAVENDER-COTTON
Satureia montana	SAVORY
Thuja occidentalis	THUJA
Thymus vulgaris	THYME
Zingiber officinale	GINGER

PART ONE

1. The Healing Power of Plants

Pour atteindre à la vérité, il faut une fois dans sa vie, se défaire de toutes les opinions que l'on a reçues, et reconstruire de nouveau et dès le fondement, les systèmes de ses connaissances.

Descartes

In my home country around Huanne I used to know an old herdsman, a cultured man in his way, whose name was Brenot. Though he died in 1940, he is still remembered in that part of Franche-Comté; it was from him I had my first lesson in the art of healing.

I was fourteen at the time and, since it was August, on holiday from school. Brenot had just come back with his herd from a pasture at Presnay near the road to Rougemont, and as usual I was waiting to help him tether the cows in their shed – a job I enjoyed. He had taught me how to avoid injury from a cow's horns by putting my chin on the creature's back, behind the ears, as I fastened the chain. He would start at one end of the cowshed, I at the other, which gave us five cows each to tie up; and if I got behind, my old friend would contrive to do the same so that he never finished before me.

That day, quite out of character, he suddenly began to curse the three-year-old heifer second from the end, Poumone, and in terms I had never heard him use before. When we emerged a few minutes later, I saw the cause of his angry outburst: almost in the centre of his right cheek was a great gash Poumone had inflicted with her horn as she turned her head. Brenot was very good at giving advice to others!

My immediate reaction was to go and look for a bottle of antiseptic or some tincture of iodine. "Don't worry," the old man said, "tomorrow there won't be anything to see." And with that, he took a piece of cobweb and applied it directly to the wound.

Next day Brenot had replaced his peculiar dressing with a thick paste made from herbs he had gathered from the side of the road leading down to the presbytery. I have an idea that plantains, and possibly walnut leaves, were involved. He had certainly been over-optimistic in predicting his cure within twenty-four hours. Nevertheless in a week the wound had healed and my friend was able to shave, as he always did, on Sunday morning before he went to mass.

Being ignorant of so much, a child often fails to be amazed by things that might reasonably deserve his astonishment. But I had heard grown-ups talking about tetanus and the dung-heap, and of all the harmful microbes found in the soil and on the horns of cattle, so that the anti-septic and cicatrising properties of the spider's web did not, after all, fail to surprise me. Of course I was completely unaware of the active consti-tuents of the plants Brenot also used. I had never heard that the walnut leaf contains an active antibiotic element which is effective against anthrax; neither had he – but he was well aware of its curative power, and that was good enough for him.[1]

Since then I have been in a position to observe hundreds of astonishing and spectacular results, and I have always found it a cause for rejoicing whenever a scientific, or at least a satisfactory, explanation has been found for observed therapeutic results, thanks to the vast body of modern experimental work which is casting increasing light on the composition and secrets of plants. It was through this kind of research that garlic was discovered to contain two antibiotic constituents which are highly effec-tive against staphylococcus, and a single clove of garlic to have sufficient antiseptic strength to preserve a side of boiled beef for twenty-four hours.

Aromatics which have the properties of phenols or aldehydes[2], such as cloves, thyme, savory and cinnamon, have traditionally been used in the everyday preparation of food, particularly in tropical countries where intestinal fermentations can assume serious forms. It is known that the essence of thyme destroys the anthrax bacillus, Eberth's bacillus (the typhoid agent), the glanders bacillus, staphylococcus, Löffler's bacillus (diphtheria), meningococcus, and Koch's bacillus (responsible for tuber-culous lesions). This has been variously demonstrated by Chamberland in 1887, Cadéac and Meunier in 1889 and Professors Courmont, Morel and Rochaix shortly before 1920. The essence of thyme has been found to have a bactericidal power stronger than that of phenol, long con-sidered the epitome of an antiseptic.

I must digress for a moment here to explain that when I call something a typhoid "agent", or Koch's bacillus "responsible for tuberculous lesions", I really intend the reader to understand that it is "encountered" in typhoid or tuberculosis. A microbe is not always the cause of an ill-ness; normally it simply bears witness to a deficiency in the organism under attack. The microbe is of far less importance than the site.

Only a small proportion of the doctors who tend patients suffering from tuberculosis or poliomyelitis contract the infection. It seems logical to infer that the victims have in fact suffered from some general lessening of resistance which has allowed Koch's bacillus or the polio virus to

1 "More than five hundred plants are made use of in Europe alone. Though some form part of the official medicine of many countries, others – and they are in the majority – have only local reputations. These may stretch back over hundreds if not thousands of years." – *Professor Perrot*

2 i.e. spices containing chiefly phenols or aldehydes which are antiseptic consti-tuents.

establish itself and multiply in their tissues. "Man brings about his illnesses by his own physiological means," said René Leriche.

In the Maquis resistance movement during the war years 1942–1945, I knew a man from Alsace whose general health was poor – in fact he had bilateral tuberculous pulmonary lesions. But his enforced stay in the open (we were out in the woods at all times of day and night) cured him of his tuberculosis without any treatment at all. One reads of severe cases of tuberculosis cured simply by the use of biological medications and essences without the slightest intervention of modern chemical or antibiotic therapy. Are sanatoria constructed in the middle of built-up areas? Of course not. They are established among pine-trees and in parts of the countryside where the air is considered particularly healthy on account of local patterns of vegetation.

Azaloux wrote: "The fact that a microbe has invaded an organism is not in itself sufficient for the infection to develop. This requires certain favourable conditions relating either to the virulence or quality of the microbes, or to the point of entry, or else to the degree of resistance of the area, i.e. the organism." Infection does not automatically follow the penetration of an organism by a microbe; the germ has to find a suitable breeding-ground.

Today great emphasis is placed on resistance. Certainly, without the natural resistance of the organism, the human race would have vanished long ago. Without going too far back into the history of epidemics, we know that the great fourteenth-century plague, so terrifying that it became known as the Black Death, carried off eighty million people in Europe alone in the space of a few years; yet mankind triumphed over it. Such slaughter might have seemed a fearful prelude to the elimination of the human species, yet not one of the peoples so decimated has disappeared. We shall see how aromatic herbs, or rather their essences, then in frequent use, played their part in this.

The extraordinary powers of the onion seem to have been known since the dawn of time. Dioscorides, a Greek doctor living in the first century AD, praised it for its diuretic and tonic properties and its effectiveness against infection. Pliny spoke of it in similar terms. But this was the extent of their knowledge, and not until many centuries later was it discovered that the juice of an onion acts as an antibiotic against staphylococcus and other microbes. Nor were its constituents known. These include iron, sulphur, iodine, silica, potassium salts, phosphates and nitrates. From this analysis we can understand more specifically how the onion has its effect. While it is true that we cannot yet explain its action on cerebral congestion, or on freckles (we are equally unable to explain the effectiveness of may-dew) we do now know why, for instance, it eases the throbbing pain of the wasp-sting so effectively. Since the work of Collip in 1923 and Laurin in 1934 we know that the onion has proved extremely valuable in cases of diabetes because of its gluconin. The work of Hull Walton, incidentally, confirms its value as an aphrodisiac, a claim of long standing.

The midwife who gave an expectant mother with a weak uterus an infusion of vervain could not know that it contained verberin, a powerful activator of uterine contractions, as Kotoku Kuwazima was to discover. Sage, a plant held sacred by the Romans, has long been used for its many properties, among which its effect in regulating and promoting menstrual periods has always been known. But the explanation for this only recently emerged with the discovery of oestrogen, a hormone which encourages the menstrual cycle in women, indeed in all female mammals. A purified extract of sage injected into mice produces effects comparable to those of folliculin. These results have been confirmed by the examination of cervical scrapes.

It comes as no great surprise that ginseng, a root used in the Far East for its tonic and aphrodisiac properties, was discovered by R. Paris to contain substances similar to folliculin. What, though, of liquorice, chiefly known for its digestive and anti-ulcerous properties, which as Costello and Lyun have shown also contains oestrogen? In an article entitled "Vegetable Hormones", which appeared in *Santé Publique* in 1961, Decaux drew attention to the need to be aware that certain vegetable substances contain sexual hormones. This knowledge is essential if one is trying to remedy hormonal insufficiencies by treatment or diet based on the use of plants. It is equally necessary if one is to avoid giving a patient an excess of hormones which might be prejudicial to his or her general health.

Decaux instances ivy as likely to produce modifications relating to the menstrual cycle in a rat whose ovaries have been removed (R. Paris and Quevauviller); again it may be remarked that the ancients knew and used ivy in the treatment of menstrual troubles. Hops also contain oestrogen, which is found in considerable quantities in beer. Could one relate to this the fact that the tissue of heavy beer drinkers is generally invaded by fat? We know of the existence of certain clovers containing oestrogen which can cause reproductive problems in sheep. In fact, as we shall see, numerous plants contain hormones: chervil, for instance; parsley, long appreciated for its emmenagogic properties, (i.e. properties which promote or regulate the menstrual cycle); water-lily, which Léon Binet calls "the destroyer of pleasure and poison to love"; willow, hollyhock, tulip . . . . One could say that the essence is to the plant as the hormones are to the endocrinal glands.

The cholagogic and choleretic properties of rosemary – that is, properties which facilitate the evacuation of bile or which increase its secretion – have been used from time immemorial. Chabrol provided proof: in an animal, the intravenous injection of an infusion of rosemary doubles the volume of bile secreted. This is just one example of the rare privilege phytotherapy and aromatherapy possess, of being at the same time the most ancient and yet the most up-to-date of therapies. For doctors and public opinion may, in recent years, have rediscovered the medicinal value of plants and aromatic essences, but the idea of using their properties to maintain or regain health goes back, as I have shown, to antiquity. "Many things will be reborn which have been long forgotten," wrote Horace.

Whilst being the oldest of all systems, phytotherapy and aromatherapy are also those which have most effectively proved themselves, fashion permitting. It might still seem strange in an age of sulphonamides, hormones and synthetic products with dazzling names which can run on for several lines, to propose as both effective and sometimes spectacular a therapeutic method based on the simple and exclusive use of plants and their essential oils. But the brief glimpse we have had so far ought surely to be sufficient to convince us of its efficacy and perennial nature. Countless cases have demonstrated its power.

Some years ago, for instance, a woman had the misfortune to upset a saucepan of boiling water over her left forearm and hand. A nurse dressed the lesions with a mixture of aromatic essences which had long seemed to me the ideal treatment for burns, its chief constituents being lavender, thyme, geranium, rosemary and sage. She completed the dressing with a bandage, simply as a precaution.

Next day the patient phoned asking to see me as quickly as possible. She wanted me to have a look at her legs, which were covered in blisters. In her understandable distraction of the previous day she had been aware only of the injury to her left arm. Now, fifteen hours after the accident, her hand and forearm were no longer a problem at all: the skin was unmarked.

At this point I began the treatment to her legs, using almost as simple a method. The blisters were lanced and compresses applied for a period of half an hour. These contained a very diluted version of the same mixture of essences, in the proportion of one teaspoon to one glass of water. The patient went home with instructions to repeat the treatment herself twice a day. Four days later she was completely cured. Moreover, she had felt no pain or discomfort from the time the treatment had begun.

A colleague of mine, not a man to waste time when it comes to forming an opinion about the curative properties of a given substance, once went ahead and deliberately burned two fingers of his left hand. He immediately treated one finger with the mixture of aromatic essences. The other he left alone. In a matter of minutes there was no pain in the treated finger, and next day not even a sign of the burn. The other finger, however, was very sore and covered in blisters, giving him ample time to observe and feel the difference. . . . Reckoning that he had now done enough in the cause of science, my colleague wrapped the finger which had been neglected for twenty-four hours in compresses soaked in the diluted form of the same preparation; again in four days the burn had healed.

Whether used fresh or in powder form, in infusions or decoctions, internally or externally by means of fumigations, liniments, poultices or baths, plants have, generally speaking, come up to expectation – so long as these important conditions are observed: they must be picked at the right moment and in a predetermined place; they must be dried and preserved skilfully so as to keep ther power intact, and they must be used with discrimination.

The medicinal use of aromatic essences – otherwise known as plant essences, essential oils or volatile oils – has a long tradition. However, in spite of a great deal of scientific investigation their method of action is still not precisely known, but this in no way diminishes their therapeutic value. In contrast to many modern medicines, with very rare exceptions, and then only when used on patients with some particular predisposition, neither plants nor their essences cause repercussions or complications – an excellent reason, if more were needed, for turning to them.

Each century has contributed its own plant recipes and prescriptions. The Egyptians embalmed their corpses with compounds containing resins and essences. Chaste Susanna took orange-flower baths in Babylon. The Greeks were familiar with perfumes, which they used for healing. The Romans grew aromatic herbs. In the Middle Ages, famous ladies had their own personal recipes . . . .

Before we make a closer study of essential oils, we might note in passing that nowadays the properties of plants and their essences are in fact used in many pharmaceutical preparations. Both doctors and housewives are behaving like M. Jourdain in Molière's *Le Bourgeois Gentilhomme* – quite unconsciously they are already practising phyto- and aromatherapy!

2. The Facts about Essential Oils

Aromatic essences are volatile, oily, fragrant substances which can be obtained from plants in a variety of ways: sometimes by *pressing* (e.g. cloves), sometimes by *tapping* (laurel, liquid Borneo camphor), sometimes by *separation* using heat (turpentine), in some cases by *solvents*, or by *enfleurage* (i.e. absorption of the perfume by a greasy substance from which it is afterwards separated).

Very often the essential oils are present-in such small quantities in comparison with the mass of the plant, and they adhere so strongly to the plants that contain them, that *distillation* of the plant is necessary. The normal method of procedure is very similar to that used in the production of distilled water; however, the same water must be distilled with further quantities of the substances, since if this is not done a considerable quantity of essence will be lost.

Certain of these essential oils do appear in the pharmacopoeiae of the world. In France, the 1949 edition – Codex VII – contains about fifteen. Earlier editions contained many more – twenty-four in 1937, forty-four in 1837[1].

Aromatic essences in general pre-exist in plants, though there are some which form only in the presence of water.

Though generally colourless, a few essences are distinctively coloured: the essence of cinnamon, for instance, is reddish, the essence of camomile, blue and the essence of wormwood, green. Some (e.g. the essences of bitter almonds, cinnamon and garlic) are heavier than water, but most are lighter. Again although most essences are liquids, some are solids.

Essences are to be distinguished from fatty oils, which are fixed and stain a paper permanently, in that they are volatised by heat and their stain is temporary. They are soluble in alcohol, ether and fixed oils and insoluble in water, to which they nevertheless impart their odour.

Their boiling points vary from 160° to 240°C, and their densities from

---

1   The requirements of the Codex demand a minimum standard of analysis of physical properties (density, solubility in alcohols of various strengths and in other solvents, boiling point, polarimetric deviation, refractive index, melting point, etc) and chemical properties (research and dosages of one of the constituents or of a combination which forms a chemical function – for example, phenols, aldehydes, alcohols, etc). To avoid overloading the present work I have mentioned only a few of these details which are generally without use to the practitioner.

0.759 to 1.096. They may be dextrorotatory or laevorotatory[2], rarely inactive, to polarised light.

They dissolve grease, iodine, sulphur and phosphorous. They reduce certain salts.

They are stimulants which can be used both internally and externally, usually in a solution of alcohol or another suitable solvent, although they can be used neat. They are also perfumes.

There was a time when essences were considered to be definite substances, but with the birth of the science of organic chemistry at the end of the nineteenth century, they gradually began to yield up their secrets – though even today all has not yet been revealed. Dr Taylor of the University of Austin, Texas has observed that essences present more new compounds than the chemists of the whole world could analyse in a thousand years. At least we now know that they are mixtures of many constituents: terpenes, alcohols, esters, aldehydes, ketones and phenols, etc. Without going into unnecessary detail here, I should add that they have been divided into three groups according to their elementary composition:.

1) *Hydrocarbon essences*, i.e. those rich in terpenes (e.g. the essences of turpentine and lemon); these are the most numerous.
2) *Oxygenised essences* (e.g. the essences of rose and mint); these are generally solid essences.
3) *Sulphuretted essences* (the Cruciferae and Liliaceae).

Many essences are a mixture of carbides and oxygenised substances in which one finds most of the chemical functions of organic matter: *hydrocarbons* or terpenes such as thymen, *alcohols* such as geraniol and linalol, *aldehydes* like the essences of bitter almonds and citral, *esters* like the acetates of bornyl and linalyl, *ketones* like carvone and thujone, and *phenols* like eugenol, thymol and carvacrol.

Some essences whose composition have been clearly defined, or at least appears to have been, are reproduced synthetically; but there are good grounds for believing that the results obtained with synthetic essences cannot be compared with the effects of natural essential oils, and practice bears this out.

The *whole* natural essence is found to be more active that its principal constituent. Moreover, those constituents which form a smaller percentage of the whole are found to be more active than the principle constituent (this is an example of synergy). As early as 1904 Cuthbert Hall demonstrated that the anti-septic properties of the essences of eucalyptus were much more powerful than those of its principal constituent, eucalyptol.

"It is not enough," wrote M. Huerre in 1919, "to place side by side the principal chemical elements which analysis shows to be present in a particular vegetable essence, in order to obtain a product which, therapeutically speaking, is as active as that of the natural essence."

2 Dextrorotatory: rotating to the right, especially rotating thus the plan of polarization of light; laevorotatory: rotating the plane of polarisation of light to the left (these characteristics are used to differentiate various bodies).

Here is a curious and apposite case. A man was being treated for a fistula of the anus by instillation of *pure and natural* drops of lavender essence. The patient had begun to recover when we went on a journey, and, discovering that he had left his essence at home, bought a fresh supply at a chemist's.

Unfortunately this essence was neither natural nor pure: one single instillation was followed by a painful inflammation of such severity that the unfortunate person was unable to sit down for more than a fortnight.

Similarly, many skin diseases and various other troubles (nervousness, dizziness, etc) follow from the use of certain perfumes and Eaux de Cologne which have been prepared from synthetic essences for the sake of economy.

These essences are often irritant to the skin. Many people, in fact, owe their troubles to using poor quality Eaux de Cologne, whose stupefacient, convulsion-inducing and allergy-forming properties are well known.

The quality of essential oils depends on many factors. The process by which a substance is obtained, its state of maturity and preservation and its source are all important. There are "prize localities" for certain essences: Ceylon, for cinnamon, the West Indies for lemongrass, Réunion for thyme, and so on.

The yield may vary from one to ten – which is to say that quality in essential oils, as in anything else, has to be paid for. Here is a table of the *average quantities* of various aromatic essences which 100kg of the relevant plant will yield.

Thyme	200g
Parsley (herb)	300g
Wormwood	300 to 400g
Hyssop	400g
Juniper	500g to 1.2kg
Valerian (root)	950g
Sage·	1.6 to 1.7kg
Ylang-ylang (flowers)	1.6 to 2kg
Lavender	2.9kg
Eucalyptus	3kg

Essential oils are often *adulterated*, with alcohol, fixed oils, essential oils of less value and certain synthetic esters such as soap from animal fat or gelatine, though there are various methods of identifying this adulteration.

Finally, I should mention here that to preserve these essences one should keep them in well-sealed containers away from the air and light (use coloured glass). It is vital to avoid oxidation, polymerisation and resinification which will occur if these precautions are not taken.

Man has a tendency to believe that what he sees is valid only for his own time. When one considers the history of aromatic essences, one may go back thousands of years to find distillation of plants being practised in ancient Persia, Turkey and India. The Romans had their knowledge of the process from the Greeks, who in their turn had received it from

Egypt. The Egyptians seem to have known how to prepare an essence of cedarwood, for instance, four thousand years ago: the wood was heated in a clay vessel with its opening covered by a screen of woollen fibres; the essence would then be obtained by squeezing out the impregnated wool.

The Arabs discovered the distilling of plants in the Middle Ages. In the thirteenth century the new pharmaceutical industry encouraged the development of distillation, and about this time the Master Glovers were granted the right to impregnate their gloves with perfume and to sell scented oils. The essence of rosemary was one of the first to be isolated at this time. In the sixteenth century the perfume industry in Provence was producing essences of lavender and aspic. It was a trade that flourished especially at Montpellier, Narbonne and Grasse.

According to Gildemeister, the aromatic essences of aspic, bitter almonds, cedar, cinnamon, frankincense, juniper, mastic, rose and sage were all known by the fifteenth century. During the next hundred years, sixty more essences came to be added to the list, and these included aloes, angelica, aniseed, basil, bay, bryony, camomile, cardamom, caraway, celery, cloves, coriander, cumin, fennel, galingale, ginger, guaiacum, hyssop, lavender, mace, melissa, myrrh, nutmeg, orange, origanum, parsley, pepper, peppermint, rue, saffron, sandalwood, savory, sassafras, sweet marjoram, tansy, thyme and wild thyme. By the beginning of the seventeenth century, with the isolation of the essences of artemisia, bergamot, box-wood, cajuput, chervil, cypress, mustard, orange-flower, pine, savin, thuja and valerian among others, most of the useful essences of Europe and the Near East had been discovered.

In France at the time of Louis XIV it was considered good form to take an interest in concoctions of essences which bore one's own name. Thus there was a powder "à la Maréchale" named after the Maréchale d'Aumont; any number of perfumes, creams and cosmetics were dressed up with the family name of one of the great lords or ladies. But the general lack of hygiene led to such an abuse of perfumes that towards the end of his reign the Sun King simply forbade them.

From the eighteenth century onwards attempts were made to control the adulteration of essential oils. This was the time when Feminis created the "eau admirable", later to be called "Eau de Cologne". A nephew, Farina, established a house in Paris to market the product.

With the nineteenth century came the first analyses. From 1818 it was well known that all terpenic hydrocarbons were in the constant proportion of five carbon atoms to eight hydrogen atoms. In 1825, Boulet discovered cumarin. Kékulé coined the name "terpene" in 1866, and the following year benzoic aldehyde was prepared for the first time by a chemical process. Perkin synthesised cumarin in 1868, and in 1876, in the rue Saint-Charles in Paris, G. de Laire founded the first factory for the synthetic prepartion of perfumes. 1822 saw the establishing of the constitution of eugenol, a fundamental element of the essence of cloves; the first artificial musk was produced in 1887. Clearly we are no longer now in the infancy of things synthetic and artificial – the first steps into the chemical era have been taken. It is precisely since that time that Western man has begun to absorb chemical colourings and preservatives with his food, and, latterly, antibiotics and synthetic hormones, substances productive of all those formidable ailments so appropriately called the "ills of civilisation" which include cardio-vascular complaints, allergies and cancer. Indeed, Professor A. Tyler, Professor of Embryology at the California Institute of Technology, has described cancer as a form of allergy. Be that as it may, it is unlikely that in future it will be chemotherapy that will provide a cure for cancer, which is a condition apparently provoked, or at least provided with favourable conditions, by a multiplicity of synthetic products.

A number of essences have established reputations; some have already acquired the patents of nobility – citral and linalol, for instance, whose composition has been studied since 1890, and other alcohols and important aliphatic aldehydes such as citronellal and geraniol. (We should note too, in another context, that 1907 saw the discovery of hydroxy-citronellal, a substance of primary importance in perfumery.)[3]

I have included this brief history to show that the chemical analysis of plants and essences goes back well over a hundred years; yet in spite of this body of research, phyto- and aromatherapy underwent a period of neglect from which, with the proliferation of present-day experimental work, they are only now emerging. Perhaps the main reason for such periods of neglect, recurrent throughout the history of plant therapy, is that every so often people will believe that they have found a panacea in some particular substance or method, and will abandon or disown everything else so long as the fashion lasts. Another explanation can be found in the matter of harvesting and preparation, for, to possess their full potentiality, plants must come from good soil, (I have already mentioned a few of the "prize localities" for certain essences)[4] must be harvested at

---

3 For those who are interested, here are the principal odoriferous products of animal origin:

a) *Ambergris.* This is a calculus formed in the digestive tract of certain large adult sperm-whales. Its prime cost, as might be imagined, is very great.

b) *Musk* is produced by the male musk-deer, which is found in the mountains of Central Asia. This animal has a pouch, situated between the navel and the sexual organs, where the odoriferous substance is secreted.

c) *Civet* perfume is provided by a carnivorous cat-like animal, the civet, found chiefly in Ethiopia, Guinea and Senegal.

d) *Castoreum* obtained from the Canadian or Siberian musquash, is the least used of these substances.
   The fumes released when ambergis, musk or castoreum are heated are said to prevent an epileptic crisis.

4 For instance, the essences produced by the different species of thyme show clear differences in chemical composition: some are essences of thymol, others of carvacrol, others again of citral (related to the essences of lemongrass).

the right moment and prepared and preserved with skill. Unfortunately, these conditions have not always been and are not always met, and this is why failure is so prevalent. Then, of course, it is the method rather than the spoilt material that tends to receive the blame. Lastly, man has always tried to base his opinions on statistics and the results of objective analyses, and by and large this is to the credit of the scientific spirit. But for a long time science failed to give this kind of explanation for the therapeutic action of plants. That phyto- and aromatherapy have recently found new favour among doctors and the general public is due to the publication of many works of scholarship on these subjects – detailed works on phytochemistry, chromatography and spectrography, X-ray examinations and various general expositions – so that, day by day, statistics are demonstrating that traditional, empirically-based notions were well-founded after all.

Surely we should be filled with admiration, and humbled too, as we discover how accurate was the information about plants and essences that the ancients possessed and how effective their application of that knowledge – more especially when we think that to reach the same point ourselves has required so much research and experimentation, often of a complex and delicate nature demanding highly sophisticated equipment. In this whole field we find, as a rule, that we can add little to what has been handed down to us. So we must recognise the fact that our forefathers were right. Goethe once wrote: "In my own canton there were wise men who could read no more than their breviary".

In the most ancient medical text of all, written 2,000 years BC, Emperor Kiwang-Ti was already studying opium, rhubarb and the pomegranate, attributing properties to them which we would not dispute today. Time and again one is made aware that the traditions of simple people include facts one did not even suspect. Take coltsfoot for example, the old wives' cough medicine: the ash contains potassium (28.23%), sodium (2.36%), calcium (21%), magnesium (8.86%), iron (1%), phosphorus (4.44%), sulphur (26.17%) and silicic acid (7.82%), making it not merely one of the most ancient effective expectorants, but also one of the best. Again, it was eventually verified that honeysuckle contains a substance with an antibiotic effect against staphylococcus and the colon bacillus – a piece of information which should endear the plant to doubting Thomases who never having cultivated the habit of observation know only how to dismiss out of hand. Or we find that the roots of the hydrangea genus contain an anti-malarial substance said to be more effective than quinine – compare this discovery with the saying that the remedy should be looked for in the same place as the disease. The forget-me-not genus, myosotis, drew the attention of Léon Binet, former Dean of the Paris Faculty of Medicine, who established among other things that it contains a large proportion of potassium (42 to 57g per kg). On this basis he recommended its use in the treatment of asthenia, hypotension, constipation and the after-effects of paralysis.

It is conceivable that the day will come when the true therapeutic value of natural substances will be given proper recognition. After all, future generations will doubtless be as non-plussed by certain theories and medical teachings that today occupy a respectable position as we are by the treatment for scabies common in the eighteenth century – blood-lettings and purges designed to aid the passage of ill-humours which "sought to escape via the skin".

3. Nature's Antiseptics

Since it was discovered that they are rich in terpenes and phenols, alcohols and aldehydes, natural essences have been regarded as necessarily endowed with *antiseptic properties*, though in fact their bactericidal action had been established in practice for thousands of years.

There is a relationship between the bactericidal power of aromatic essences and their chemical function: in order of decreasing potency we have phenols, aldehydes, alcohols, esters and acids (opinions still differing with regard to the terpenes). These constituents generally have greater antiseptic properties than synthetic phenol, long used as a reference. The Medical School at Lyons, for example, has shown that the minimum concentrations needed to ensure complete absence of fertilisation[1] of Koch's bacillus are: of eugenol 0.05 per thousand, thymol 0.1 per thousand, guaiacol 0.8 per thousand, phenol 0.8 per thousand.

Since the *chemical* nature of the essences is very variable, while their antiseptic power is general, it is thought that this property common to essences must be attributed to common physical properties. Some authors hold that the disinfectant action of essences is proportional to a reduction in the surface tension[2]; others that it is attributable to special solubility on the limiting film of living cells.

The antiseptic power has been determined both in the presence of essence vapours and in direct contact with essential oils.

The first research into the antiseptic powers of essential oils was undertaken by Chamberland in 1887, in his work on the anthrax bacillus. He noted the active properties of origanum, Chinese cinnamon, Singhalese cinnamon, angelica and Algerian geranium.

The *antigenetic*[3] potency of essences in their vapourised state appears in the following decreasing order: lemon, thyme, orange, bergamot, juniper, clove, citronella, lavender, niaouli, peppermint, rosemary, sandalwood, eucalyptus, Chinese anise. This order corresponds almost exactly with the strength of essences studied in respect of their terpenes.

1 Action which impedes the development of microbial cultures.
2 Strength present if the surface-film of liquids which by reason of a particular arrangement of molecules acquires properties analogous to those of an elastic membrane.
3 i.e. which combats the development of germs and kills them.

The antigenetic potency of these vapours is experienced above all in relation to meningococcus, staphylococcus and the typhus bacillus. The diphtheric bacillus is much more strongly resistant, and the spores of the anthrax bacillus are not affected at all.

The decreasing order of antigenetic activity in essential oils is slightly different in the case of direct contact: thyme, lemon, juniper, peppermint, niaouli, eucalyptus, sandalwood, anise, Chinese anise.

Cavel's research on microbic cultures in sewage has shown many essences to have infertilising properties at considerable dilutions. In decreasing order of activity, for a thousand parts of microbic culture, the following essences have shown themselves effective in these proportions: essence of thyme, 0.7; of origanum, one part in a thousand; of lemongrass, 1.6; of rose, 1.6; cinnamon, 1.7; cloves, two parts in a thousand; eucalyptus 2.25; peppermint and geranium, 2.5; meadowsweet 3.3; aspic 3.5; aniseed and mustard 4.2; birch, 4.8. I think one must admit that this list has already yielded some surprises.

Cavel's results have been correlated. The following table shows in cubic centimetres the minimum dose of various essences that will render infertile 1000cc of meat stock cultured in septic tank water:

Essence	Dose rendering infertile per 1000cc
Thyme	0.7
Origanum	1.0
Sweet Orange	1.2
Lemongrass	1.6
Chinese cinnamon	1.7
Rose	1.8
Clove	2.0
Eucalyptus	2.25
Peppermint	2.5
Rose Geranium	2.5
Meadowsweet	3.3
Aspic	3.5
Chinese anise	3.7
Orris	3.8
Cinnamon (Singhalese)	4.0
Wild Thyme	4.0
Anise	4.2
Mustard	4.2
Rosemary	4.3
Cumin	4.5
Neroli (orange flower)	4.75
Birch	4.8
Lavender	5.0
Melissa (Balm)	5.2
Ylang-ylang	5.6

Juniper (berries)	6.0
Sweet fennel............................	6.4
Garlic..................................	6.5
Lemon	7.0
Cajuput	7.2
Sassafras...............................	7.5
Heliotrope.............................	8.0
Turpentine.............................	8.6
Parsley	8.8
Violet	9.0

In comparison, the infertilising quantity of phenol, fixed in identical conditions, was 5.6 per thousand.

In a very diluted alcoholic solution (between 2% and 7%), the essences of palmarosa, cinnamon and cloves in particular were found to be active with regard to homogenous cultures of the tuberculosis bacillus (Courmont, Morel and Rochaix, Morel and Bay).

The essences of eucalyptus, cloves, niaouli, thyme, garlic, sandalwood, lemon, cinnamon, lavender, German camomile and peppermint are particularly notable for their antiseptic properties, and some of these, I think, deserve to be singled out for closer attention.

The essences of eucalyptus is sometimes replaced by its chief constituent, eucalyptol, This substance is used in an oily solution (5 to 10 g %) as a nasal application and is also given in intra-muscular injections. Internally, it is administered in 0.2g capsules. Some researchers, however, give the leading role to the terpenic carbides which eucalyptus contains, and to them eucalyptol appears to be a lifeless substance.

The essence of cloves kills the tuberculosis bacillus at a strength of one part to six thousand. In dentistry it is used as a disinfectant and cauterising agent, though for this purpose it is being increasingly replaced by its principal constituent, eugenol. The antiseptic power of the essence is such that even if used in a 1% dilution, it is still 3 to 4 times more active than phenol.[4]

4 It is worth remembering the recent discovery of a new, safe narcotic anaesthetic in West Germany. For up until this time the use of all narcotics and anaesthetics required the accompanying use of preventive injections of another medicament in order to avoid complications; it was also necessary to make sure that the patient had previously fasted for a considerable time. A new narcotic obtained from cloves makes these preparations unnecessary. There is a complete absence of vomiting at the end of a period of narcosis, even if the patient has eaten shortly before the operation. This is particularly significant when an operation has to be performed urgently, as in the case of a road accident. Similarly, the danger of respiratory arrest which always exists with other narcotics is removed: far from lowering the rate of respiration, an injection of the new substances actually increases it. The state of torpor resulting from the use of other rapid narcotics is likewise avoided. Fifteen to twenty minutes after the operation the patient is entirely lucid.

The essence of niaouli is used in a 5 to 10% oily solution, to soothe wounds, burns or ulcers. Niaouli water is also used, in a 2% solution.[5] It is prepared by shaking, and is taken internally in the form of capsules of niaouli at 50% (1g per day). Niaouli has traditionally been used in New Caledonia, its inhabitants eating the leaves, making infusions and using the essence to disinfect water.

The essence of thyme is an excellent antiseptic, obviously on account of the thymol it contains. Much has been written on the bactericidal power of the peroxidised essence (i.e. the essence oxidised to a higher degree) at a strength of 1.5%. The aqueous solution at 5% kills the typhus bacillus (typhoid fever) and Shiga's bacillus (agent of epidemic dysentery) in 2 minutes. It can kill the colon bacillus in 2–8 minutes, streptococcus and the diphtheric bacillus in 4 minutes, staphylococcus in 4–8 minutes and the tuberculosis bacillus in 30–60 minutes. At a strength of 0.1%, the peroxidised essence of thyme in a diluted solution of soapy water destroys the mouth's microbial flora within 3 minutes.

The essence of garlic is used in a preventive capacity during influenza epidemics, and as a modifier of bronchial secretions.

The essence of sandalwood is a specific for the disinfection of the urinary tract, generally taken in capsules of 0.25g. Other essences are also powerful urinary disinfectants, in particular juniper, lavender and turpentine.

The essence of lemon is second to none in its antiseptic and bactericidal properties. The works of Morel and Rochaix have demonstrated that the *vapours* of lemon essence neutralise the meningococcus in 15 minutes, the typhus bacillus in less than an hour, pneumococcus in 1–3 hours, *Staphylococcus aureus* in 2 hours and haemolytic streptococcus in 3–12 hours. The *essence* itself neutralises the typhus bacillus and staphylococcus in 5 minutes and the diphtheric bacillus in 20 minutes. A few drops of lemon will rid an oyster of 92% of its micro-organisms in 15 minutes (Ch. Richet).

The essence of German camomile has a constituent called azulene with surprising bacteriostatic properties. At a strength of 1 part to 2000, it is efficacious against *Staphylococcus aureus*, haemolytic streptococcus (agent of scarlet fever and acute rheumatoid arthritis), and the *Proteus vulgaris*. Infected wounds have been healed using a concentration of between 1 to 85,000 and 1 to 170,000.

The antiseptic properties of the essences of cinnamon, peppermint and lavender are described in separate sections. I shall mention here simply that *the essence of cinnamon* will kill the typhus bacillus in a dilution of 1 part in 300.

I have described the bactericidal powers of vaporised lemon essence: Professor Griffon, Director of the French Police Toxicology Laboratory and member of the Academy of Pharmacy and of the Higher Council for Hygiene, studied the antiseptic effect of a blend of aromatic essences –

---

5 The 2% solution (2g of essence to 1 litre of water) seems, for many essences, to be the most suitable.

pine, thyme, peppermint, lavender, rosemary, cloves and cinnamon – in the *bacteriological purification of the air.*

The research was conducted in collaboration with the Veterinary Health Service of Paris and the Seine, as he acknowledges in his report, dated 7th January 1963.

The mixture of essences was sprayed from an aerosol. Professor Griffon studied the virulence of the microscopic germs present in the air before and after exposure to the spray, the germs being collected as they settled in open Petri dishes.[6]

The results can be summarised as follows: 15cm from ground-level (where microbic multiplication is most important – much more so than at 60cm, 1 metre and above) the Petri dishes, which had stood open for 24 hours in a room not yet treated with the atomizer, revealed a total of 210 colonies of microscopic flora, of which 12 were moulds and 8 staphylococci. Even after only 15 minutes the dishes already held more than 62 colonies altogether, including 8 moulds and 6 staphylococci. However, 15 minutes after the room had been treated with the spray of aromatic essences, the open dishes showed a total of only 14 colonies of microbes with 4 moulds and no staphylococci; after 30 minutes the figures were found to be 4, 0 and 0 respectively. In half an hour, therefore, the aromatic essences had destroyed all the moulds and all the staphylococci in the surrounding atmosphere, leaving only 4 microbial colonies out of an original 210.

Professor Griffon concluded that *"the atmospheric dispersion of the prepared liquid"* brought about a very marked disinfection of the air, as demonstrated by the considerable reduction in the number of pre-existing micro-organisms, some types being destroyed completely.

Already in 1960 Dr Bidault had recognised the main therapeutic role which he assigned to this preparation in the prevention of infectious childhood diseases (whooping cough, coryza or nasal catarrh, influenza) and of acute or chronic diseases of the respiratory tract in adults (influenza, tuberculosis and pneumonia). He confirmed the experiments demonstrating the germicidal action of the aromatic essences on the Bordet-Geugon bacillus (whooping cough), the Pfeiffer bacillus (influenza) and Koch's bacillus (tuberculosis).

His clinical observations proved that the disinfection of the air surrounding the patient has a therapeutic preventative effect. This evidence cannot be ignored if we consider the following facts: 5 pathogenic organisms may be found in 1 cubic metre of the Forest of Fontainbleau – 20,000 in a Paris flat, 9 million at the Motor Show and nearly as many in the big stores; a work-table has 5 million microbes per square metre, a

6   Petri dishes are made of two hollow glass discs that fit one on top of the other, like a round box and lid. A gelatine meat broth is poured into the lower disc for culturing the colonies of microbes to be studied.

carpet 9 million. In a large hospital there are on average 10,000 per cubic metre. Many years ago a doctor put some of this air into a flask containing a few drops of aromatic essences: 40% of the microbes were destroyed in 20 minutes, 80% in an hour, and in 9 hours 100%.

The administering of essential oils by fine aerosol spray should be common practice in sick rooms, operating theatres and clinics. However, since certain substances in the spray can sometimes cause allergic reactions, it is still perhaps preferable to let the essences escape into the atmosphere naturally. For the past fifteen years I have been using a small heated lamp with a crucible above it for this purpose. Into this crucible several drops of the natural essences of thyme, lavender, pine and eucalyptus are poured daily.

It was in 1949 that Professor Jean Barbaud presented his thesis on aerosols to the Academy of Pharmacy.[7] He demonstrated that the sprays made by atomisation under pressure were formed of droplets of different sizes, and that after a certain interval the heaviest particles sank to the bottom to leave an ultra-fine mist which was more homogenous. This finding justified the use of "expansion" chambers within the aerosol apparatus where the spray would be stabilised by the deposition of the heaviest particles. It would be interesting to study the possible influence of the diameter of the sprayed particles on their effectiveness both in disinfecting the surrounding air and in medical treatments.

The astonishing antiseptic power of aromatic essences is a well-established fact – we can find it recognised in such an everyday product as toothpaste, where the efficacy of anise, cloves, camomile, peppermint and other essential oils as a base is undisputed. Even the addition of the best-known bactericidal agents has done nothing to increase the antiseptic power of toothpaste made from these essences, so that it is quite understandable that, rather than using chemical products which may be dangerous or inactive against germs, manufacturers will time and again choose natural essences. Or again, in the treatment of specific diseases, if we take the tuberculosis bacillus, Professors Courmont, Morel and Rochaix have demonstrated that the active bactericidal dose is 0.1% for thymol (principal constituent of thyme oil), 0.05% for eugenol (principal constituent of clove oil) and 0.4% for essence of peppermint, whereas phenol and guaiacol are effective only at a dose of 0.8%.

In their practical applications, the essences of lemon, lavender, aspic and hyssop at 0.2%, and the essences of sweet marjoram, orange and niaouli at 0.4% prove also more effective than guaiacol and phenol. The essence of thyme has an antiseptic and antiparasitic power considerably greater than those of guaiacol, hydrogen peroxide and potassium permanganate. Further proof that the antiseptic power of aromatic essences generally equals or even surpasses that of most synthetic products may be found in a work written by Professor Sauvat of the École Nationale Vétérinaire at Toulouse in 1951, in which he observes that "the bacteri-

---

7   Jean Barbaud: On the heterogeneity of medicinal aerosols produced by atomisation under pressure.

cidal power of quaternary ammonium salts is considerably augmented when used in association with terpineol".

Some essences have been found to complement the action of antibiotics. Laboratory tests have shown that, for instance, even the purified essence of niaouli (gomenol) will increase the activity of streptomycin and, more especially, of penicillin (Quevauviller and Parousse-Perrin, *Revue de Pathologie Comparée*, 1958). Reporting the results obtained when using turpentine derivatives in conjunction with antibiotics, Mignon has shown, from tests "in vitro" and on mice, the action of the antibiotics to be considerably augmented by being administered in a solution of oxygenated turpentine derivatives. There are, however, some constituents of some essential oils (aldehydes, ketones and some alcohols) which inactivate antibiotics and so limit their use in ointment form.

In 1938, the *Belgian Tuberculosis Review* published an article by Ch. Mayer describing the testing, on guinea-pigs, of an anti-tuberculosis vaccine consisting of bacillary emulsions treated with essential oils. Fr. de Potter of the Institute of Hygiene and Bacteriology in Ghent, inspired by this account, made a study[8] of the bactericidal action of solutions on cultures of the non spore[9]-forming germs staphylococcus aureus, the typhus bacillus, the colon bacillus and the bacillus foecalis alcaligene, and the spore-forming bacillus subtilis. He used a 5% solution of geraniol, borneol and cypress.

Although the culture of the bacillus subtilis remained unaffected by the solution even after two days' exposure, at 37°C the staphylococci emulsions became sterilised in 1–2 hours, and at room temperature in 4–5 hours. The cultures of the typhus, colon and foecalis bacilli were sterilised in 20–30 minutes at 37°C and in 30–60 minutes at room temperature. A subcutaneous injection of 1 to 2cc of the solution did not cause any local painful reaction in either guinea-pig, rabbit or man, and an intravenous injection of 10cc was well tolerated by man and rabbit. Furthermore, the solution retained its bactericidal properties after being kept at a temperature of 105°C for 20 minutes, and its disinfectant properties proved superior to those of phenol.

A few months later, the same author published a study on immunisation against the staphylococcus in man and guinea-pig, using a vaccine made from an aqueous solution of essential oils. His conclusion was that such a solution made a preferable medium for the vaccine "because of its rapid and effective sterilising action without recourse to heating". For Fr. de Potter, its practical value recommended this method of preparing vaccine above other methods.

Attempts have been made to concentrate the essential oils in certain apparently highly active products by means of the processes of deterpenation and peroxidation in particular, in order to improve their antiseptic powers. Deterpination involves the separating of first the oxygenated

8 Fr. de Potter: on the bactericidal action of aqueous solutions of essential oils (*C. R. Soc. Biologie*, 1939).

9 *Spore* – the name given to the reproductive cells of certain plants, cryptogams (mushroom, fern etc) and microbes; spores can resist harsh external conditions.

constituents (phenols, alcohols, ketones, aldehydes and esters) and secondly the hydrocarbons (turpentine, sesquiturpentine) from the oils, the extraction of the hydrocarbons – usually by fractionate distillation – always proving a very delicate operation. The process gives highly variable results because of the variation in the carbide turpentine content of the different essences – lemon essence, to take one example, gives 5kg of deterpenised essence from an initial 100kg of essential oil.[10]

Experiments have indicated that deterpenation does result in an increased antiseptic action in the essential oil. This claim would appear to contradict the view mentioned above, that the antigenetic power of many essential oils in vapour form appears to correspond to their richness in turpentines.[11]

In contrast to the integral natural essences, which are almost insoluble in water and barely soluble in alcohol, the deterpenised essences are soluble in alcohol even when the strength is reduced (75° or even as low as 70° or 60°). A property more valuable still is their capability of easily dissolving non-deterpenated essences or their various constituents. These characteristics naturally give them pride of place in a number of preparations where there is a mixture of essential oils or their constituents.

The process of peroxidation involves oxidising (oxygenating) the essential oils. The turpentine derivatives can stabilise some of the oxygen which they give off under certain conditions. Researchers have hoped to increase the bactericidal action of essential oils by this method, but at present results have been inconclusive and further research has proved necessary.

In the past, when the composition of essential oils was a mystery, even without understanding the chemical processes involved people were able to profit from their antiseptic properties whether in the form of food (garlic, onion, etc) or vapours for the prevention and control of epidemics. Hippocrates, for instance, tackled the plague epidemic in Athens by fumigating the city with aromatic essences. In the nineteenth century, perfumery workers always showed an almost complete immunity during cholera outbreaks. This was forgotten in 1970 when panic raged throughout the Western world at the news of a few cases of cholera in the Near East. Because of our present-day theories, anyone leaving for black Africa or the Near East had to be vaccinated, some becoming so ill as a result that they were forced to cancel their trips. But some businessmen who escaped vaccination returned hale and hearty from the countries in question, where there was a real risk of catching this fatal disease; all they had taken with them were charcoal tablets, magnesium – and essential

10   This explains the marked strength of deterpenated essences, which is always much greater than that of the corresponding essential oil in its natural state.

11   This means that some researchers believe that essential oils owe their bactericidal power to their turpentine content while others believe that their antiseptic power is increased by deterpenation. It should be noted, however, that some studies are discussing in terms of vaporised essences, others in terms of the oils themselves and in either case the experiments refer to different categories of microbe. Until further research clarifies the situation, we shall continue to refer to the total essential oil.

oil drops. And so, to repeat Léon Binet's observation, modern research again "confirms the validity of traditional ideas based on practical experience".

In 1958, we learned that vapours derived from aromatic plants possess antiseptic properties which inhibit the development of certain staphylococci and coliform bacilli. These plants include (in descending order of potency) thyme, rosemary, eucalyptus, peppermint, orange blossom, maize, poplar, pine, Indian hemp, tobacco, belladonna, datura, henbane, hop and poppy.

The antiseptic properties of aromatic essences are put to good use every day by the housewife who uses garlic, thyme, lemon, cloves and other spices, in her kitchen[12].

The doctor who is familiar with essential oils can use them to treat a whole range of infections – pulmonary, hepatic, intestinal, urinary, uterine, rhinopharyngeal and cutaneous (infected wounds and suppurating dermatoses). The use of these oils usually produces satisfactory results, provided that they have been prescribed wisely and that, in the case of certain long-standing chronic complaints, the treatment is followed for a long enough period. Aromatic therapy can neutralise enteritis, colitis and putrid fermentations, and can relieve chronic bronchitis and pulmonary tuberculosis. The colon bacillus cannot resist essential oils. Among other medications, aromatherapy is also indicated for cancer, a complaint which is receiving a great deal of attention at the moment.[13]

Doctor Maurice Girault, a gynaecological and obstetric surgeon from Dijon, conducted over a period of six years some interesting experiments

12 *Aromatic condiments* also owe their digestive or carminative properties to their essences, and these include cinnamon, cloves, anise, cumin, chervil, parsley, mace, vanilla, tarragon, saffron, bay, savory, rosemary and thyme. When used in reasonable quantities they are quite easily tolerated by the digestive system.

Alliaceous condiments include garlic, spring onion, chives, shallots, mustard and horseradish; these can sometimes be irritant to the digestive tract.

Spicy condiments include, among others, pepper, ginger and pimento. Since pepper stimulates the digestive glands, it is suitable for patients with digestive problems. These condiments can, however, be irritant to the gastric lining, and according to a recent study, pepper, mustard and ginger have a tendency to cause high blood pressure.

13 The annual review of the American Cancer Society, published in Washington, states that more than 1,000,000 Americans living in the USA at the present time have been cured of cancer. The review adds that a further 700,000 who have been diagnosed as suffering from cancer and who have been receiving treatment over the past five years will soon be considered as cured. A cure is only classified as definitive when five years have followed the completion of the treatment without a relapse (*Sciences Techniques*, 1962). In fact, the problem is more complex than this, for some cancer patients considered cured at the end of the five-year period have died from that very disease within another two or three years, which suggests that this test ought perhaps to be reviewed. Conversely, other cancer patients who have been given only a few months to live are still alive twelve years later. They have benefitted from "alternative medicines" (*Docteur-Nature* by Jean Valnet, publ. Fayard, Paris 1971).

relating to phyto- and aromatherapy. He was convinced of the frequently harmful effects of regularly prescribed hormones, synthetic corticoids and antibiotics which it seemed to him were dispensed far too freely and in excessively high doses, and decided to make a systematic study of the effect of plants and essential oils in gynaecology, particularly in respect of the circulation and the endocrine glands, and the general restoration of physiological and nervous equilibrium, and also their anti-infectious properties.

The results of Dr Girault's experiments have been set out in scientific publications. The evidence he presented was impressive enough to undermine the scepticism of colleagues, pharmacists and, especially, the heads of test laboratories who had heard of his research. A 90% success rate cannot easily be discounted. His study of the anti-infectious, bacteri-cidal and antibiotic[14] properties of aromatic essences in the treatment of vaginal discharge constituted a considerable achievement from the point of view of both its purely scientific value and the number and quality of the cures affected. Furthermore, he availed himself, quite rightly, of the services of the best laboratories.

Dr Girault's technique was classic: first of all a swab was taken of the vaginal secretions, and their pH value[15] calculated. The microbes were then identified and placed in cultures, and finally "antibiograms" were drawn up, using essential oils or particular plant extracts. This process may be compared to the synthesis of antibiotics. For those unfamiliar with the term, an antibiogram involves the bringing together in the laboratory, in whatever culture medium is chosen, of the agents respons-ible for an infection and a number of therapeutic substances (natural or chemical). It can then be seen how effective the different substances are in dealing with the germs in question. For all its imperfection – which is inherent in the fact that only the microbe-antibiotic reaction is being studied, the third element in the drama, namely the patient, being totally ignored – this method has a certain practical usefulness.

It should be borne in mind, however, that a well-known and neatly classified microbe is not necessarily indentical to its homologue har-boured by a different host. For instance, the colibacillus present in one patient may respond to the essential oil of pine and in another patient to lavender or thyme. Individual treatment, then, is of prime importance. We must condemn, by definition, conveyor-belt medicine, which is often nothing more than a harmless routine and can sometimes be a harmful one. By the same token we deny that there is any usefulness in the hap-hazard prescriptions of the thousands of tablets which are churned out today. With the backing of his findings, Dr Girault treats his own patients with those plants and essences which he has proved to be the most active (when ingested, or taken in the form of capsules) and at the same time devoid of any harmful side-effects.

To be able to act according to his conscience, a doctor must find what today has become a rare bird – the chemist with a love of his calling. To

14   Apart from certain minor differences, these terms are comparable.
15   The degree of acidity or alkalinity, which conditions a number of infections.

qualify for this description, a chemist must be prepared to let his cosmetics and his electrical counters take care of themselves to give him time for his real job: to procure for his customers everything exactly as the doctor has prescribed – even that little packet of herb tea whose price may be derisory. Most large and some smaller towns have at least one such chemist, though I still receive letters from colleagues who, having failed to find one for themselves who is not simply a "commercial distributor of luxury articles or chemical products with an automatic sale", ask me for the name of a reliable man in Paris or elsewhere. I have little trouble in providing what they ask, for such chemists do exist – though, out of the 16,000 or so chemists in France today, they can be counted in double figures.

There are a variety of ways in which essential oils can be administered: internally, singly or in combination, and generally as pills, or drops in an alcoholic solution; externally chiefly as fumigations, inhalations, liniments and general or localised baths.[16]

Some soaps can emulsify essential oils, and the resulting preparations are obviously extremely useful for bathing wounds, and where moist dressings are needed in the treatment of boils, abscesses, lymphangitis, burns, gangrenous or cancerous wounds and leg ulcers. These emulsions could certainly be used too as vaginal injections in the treatment of many cases of hysteritis (uterine inflammation) and leucorrhea. Their germ-killing and healing action has been shown highly superior to that of oxygenated water, formalin, or Dakin's liquor, the common treatment today for suppurating wounds.[17] The aromatic substances which become soluble in water by means of a suitable "softener" may be used in the same way.

16   Certain recent scientific methods (using radio-active isotopes) have provided proof of the skin's absorption of the active principles of minerals and vegetables added to baths and later found in the blood. This discovery explains the action of the aromatic baths – for instance baths containing the essences of thyme or pine needles – on the lungs, i.e. generally antiseptic, fluidifying the mucus and aiding expectoration. Such baths certainly do have an effect through inhalation of vapour, but it is also achieved through the intermediary of the blood as the essences follow the path from the skin to the lungs.
Aromatic essential oils are among the most effective bath additives. Many studies have shown the transformations which may be caused in this way, both physically and psychologically, by their acting upon the nervous system, the alimentary canal and the urinary tract, and their hormonal action. These effects which result from the extraordinary diffusibility of the essences, suggest a logical explanation for the ancient practice of hanging a little bag of garlic cloves round the necks of children with worms, or of wearing such a bag as a protection against epidemic diseases. I mentioned earlier the outstanding diuretic properties of onion juice; turning to the past, again, we find a common method of bringing about diuresis consisted of applying poultices of onions to the kidneys and lower abdomen.

17   Carrel's method, well-known to war-time surgeons, consists in irrigating the wounds or natural cavities with a solution of Dakin's liquor, a mixture of bleach and disinfectant whose caustic effects have been neutralised with bicarbonate of soda.

Essential oils are especially valuable as antiseptics because their aggression towards microbial germs is matched by their total *harmlessness to tissue* – one of the chief defects of chemical antiseptics is that they are likely to be as harmful to the cells of the organism as to the cause of the disease. Azaloux rightly points out in his thesis [18] that "that is the real problem: to find an antiseptic which will destroy the microbes without harming the organism which is their accidental host . . . In fact, the living tissue cells intervene, reacting simultaneously to the action of both the microbe and the antiseptic." It is very important to remember that antiseptics will destroy not only the micro-organisms but also the surrounding cells. It would clearly be ridiculous to try and disinfect the entire human organism, for any substance circulating in the blood in sufficient quantity to guarantee the destruction of all bacteria would cause serious damage to the cells – and would indeed prove lethal. All chemical antiseptics irritate cells and tissue to a greater or lesser degree according to their general toxicity.

Discussing the treatment of wounds during the First World War, Azaloux observes that antiseptic irrigation was found to be not merely useless but even harmful in its effects:

> "Delbet, Fiessinger and Policard in particular established that in wounds dressed according to the Carrel method, microbes continued to persist after the end of the treatment. They showed that wounds which at the outset contained only a very few microbes, after three, four or six days contained in fact quite a large number. They also established that after forty-eight hours,the sponge tissue surrounding Carrel's tubes in wounds irrigated with this solution, was filled with microbes – more in fact than on the surface of the wound."

For this reason Delbet recommended a solution with a magnesium chloride base as a dressing, and published the results of many tests which showed its remarkable cicatrising effects. It is also one of the reasons why I myself prefer to use preparations based on aromatic essences when treating wounds, sores or burns. The seriousness of poisoning caused by the body's resorption of substances produced by degeneration of tissue and microbial toxins is well-known, so that one of the chief ways in which essences prove their superiority in the treatment of infected wounds and burns must surely be their ability to generate derivatives which, combining chemically with the substances produced by the breaking down of tissual albumins, for *atoxic* bodies, which are then eliminated from the organism.

The odour of essential oils does not *cover up* the bad smells of infected gangrenous or cancerous wounds; it suppresses them by physico-chemical action. Thus the resins and essences used in the embalming of bodies *prevent* putrefaction; the Egyptians knew it and butchers still do, for they mostly use aromatics to prevent their meat rotting.

There seem to be two major types of biological reaction: synthesis,

18   Toulouse, 1943.

whose processes give rise to forms generally characterised by sweet aromas, and degradation, whose processes are generally characterised by offensive – and in the case of rotten meat and eggs, for instance, repulsive – smells. Illness is a process of degradation which precedes décomposition, and here aromatic essences have their use in that they can hinder this process while promoting the decomposition, digestion and neutralisation of germs.

Surely this is the key factor: the antiseptic power of essences does not diminish nor become blunted with the passing of time. Why not? It is hard to find a satisfactory answer, but perhaps it is because these natural substances, besides jugulating infections, reinforce the organism's own defence mechanisms. They are in fact powerful alteratives. Furthermore, the organism does not appear to become accustomed to aromatherapy in the way that it does to synthetic sleeping pills, for instance, or – in the case of both body and germs – to the many forms of treatment using antibiotics.

Antibiotics are certainly powerful weapons, but they can be dangerous and are easily and often misused. In his book *Médecine Practicienne* Fari has detailed his own understanding of the problem they present and the *tolerance* to germs which they acquire increasingly with frequent use. In his opinion, the trouble lies in their mode of operation: antibiotics act by modifying the chemical constitution of the microbes, so that the antibodies[19] the organism produces for its own defence will be effective only against a *modified* germ.

They are therefore only "false antibodies", impotent against the real agent of infection, the germ in its original state. In showing that an antibiotic is capable of prompting an organism to manufacture these false antibodies, Fari has provided an explanation for facts which have become so widely-known as to be considered banal and indeed tiresome to reiterate. To put it plainly, the cure of an illness by means of antibiotics is a chancy business, less reliable in fact than natural recovery itself which leaves the patient strengthened against any new infection.

Many books have been written arguing the relative merits of the various synthetic medications available, and of the constant and often astonishing power of natural methods. There can be no entirely safe routine prescription of a sulphonamide drug, of an antibiotic of whatever kind, or of a synthetic hormone. "If we want the truth, then we must turn to nature," wrote Léon Binet, advocating a return to healthy habits and natural treatments under the following headings: personal hygiene and exercise, a biologically sound diet, and the observance of the natural rhythms of day and season. He also emphasised the importance of knowing the multiple properties of plants and how these may be used. The fact

19 *Antibody* – the name given to certain substances which appear in the serum of an animal or man in response to the injection of a foreign substance (whether microbes or various other elements). Some antibodies exist spontaneously in serum; these are the defence agents of the organism, their role being principally to agglutinate, dissolve or neutralise microbes or their toxins.

is that, *upheld by modern scientific research*, treatments with herbs and aromatic essences must no longer be thought comparable with the whim of some great lady indulging in a pastoral idyll.

The aromatogramme
This is an antibiogramme in which essential oils are used.

For those who do not know what an antibiogramme is, it consists of bringing together on selected culture media in a laboratory the offending infectious agents and a number of different substances (both chemical and natural) in order to ascertain the degree of effectiveness of the different products on the germs in question.

The study of the suppression of germs by aromatic oils *in vitro* was not of course discovered yesterday and many authors, such as Professors Courmont, Morel, Rochaix, Perrot, Bay, Davaine and, nearer home, Pellecuer in Montpellier – whose recent works on savory have been most useful to us – have shown to what extent oils work in minute concentrations.

When we resumed the work begun many years ago, following our findings, we decided to use this test which we called the *aromatogramme* in our daily routine.

The process involves testing various aromatic oils on germs isolated by the culture method, from a liquid or piece of organic material taken from a sick person. To do this, you pour some agar into a Petri dish and place on it some discs impregnated with oils.

Then you sub-culture the germ in the usual media for 24 hours – long enough for the culture to develop and fill the Petri dish – which is what actually happens, except in the areas occupied by the oils which have an inhibitive action on the germ. The scale runs from 0 to 3 according to the diameter of the area affected by the inhibitors and the result is expressed, as in the case of an antibiogramme, according to the degree of sensitivity of the germ to the oil.

For this test to be valid it had to satisfy the two principal criteria required by a laboratory examination: a high degree of reliability and the ability to be faithfully reproduced. Lastly, to be viable its cost had to be kept down. We established its reliability by applying multiple aromatogrammes to the same germ and we always got exactly the same results.

Its reproducibility was studied in the same way, by re-seeding the same germ at intervals of several days: there again we obtained the same results. Another way of proving its reproducibility is to conduct repeated aromatogrammes on germs taken from the same organic medium of the same patient after inadequate treatment to eradicate the germ. In such cases the variations are either slight or non-existent.

To obtain this result, a certain number of precautions were mandatory owing to the oils' two major characteristics – *qualities* therapeutically speaking but *drawbacks* from the conservation angle: their diffusibility and their volatitily.

Their volatility presented an overall conservation problem, namely how to keep the discs in an environment saturated in oils and in the dark so as to prevent oxidation by light.

Their diffusibility necessitated a reduction in the number of discs per Petri dish in order to eliminate interferences, which resulted in an increase in the cost of the test. But by reducing the concentration of oils on each disc, it was possible to retain six to eight discs per Petri dish and thus to bring the cost of the aromatogramme down to a level comparable to that of the antibiogramme.

This idea of reducing the aromatic concentration of the discs leads us straight to that of minimal active concentration on the germs. This is very important when one knows the doses we use in therapeutics and, as a result, the concentrations in the tissues.

The minimal effective concentrations are very low. Thus, Professors Courmont, Morel and Rochaix have shown that in the case of the tuberculosis bacillus, if the neutralising dose of phenol was 8 per 10,000, it was only 4:10,000 of essence of mint, 1:10,000 of thyme and 0.5:10,000 of cloves; and we have selected the case of a particularly resilient bacillus. Professor Pellecuer has recently shown that savory acted on most germs in doses half those of thyme (the effect of which we have seen to be very weak anyway), lavender and cloves.

In addition to their antibiotic effects, oils react to a *change of locality*. From a distance this phenomenon seems to us to be the most important one for, by changing the ecological conditions which made possible the development and pathogenic growth of the germs, the oils stand in the way of their survival by preventing the body from building up resistances or adapting to the attacking agent. Better still, they protect against the return of the germs, both in the short and long term.

Finally, the last advantage is that they present very little risk to the cells that will survive once the balance has been restored. In fact, as all living cells share the same method of reproduction, the counter measures usually prescribed cannot fail to have a harmful effect on the host, and fast.

So, the aromatogramme will have enabled us to adjust our anti-infection treatment by providing an important nosological element relative to the constants of the locality in which the germs developed. Indeed, it has been possible to establish that germs which flourish in a diabetic will be particularly sensitive to hypoglycemic oils. In the case of an arthritic or a gout sufferer, hypouricemic oils are the most active.

This shows quite clearly the usefulness of the aromatogramme in detecting latent pathological states in their early stages.

Apart from these oils with *localised action*, there are some which act primarily on the *functions* which govern our general state of health and which are often the first to suffer from the pace of modern life:
  – the supnarenal glands are stimulated by savory
  – the central nervous system by lavender, thyme and aspic

47

– the genital organs and libido by cinnamon, cajuput and cloves
– the intestines, the seat of so many troubles, by cinnamon, cloves and rosemary.

Finally, one can select them according to their primary *healing powers*, such as those oils which act in the region of the lungs: niaouli, eucalyptus and pine, or on the urinary system: juniper and sandalwood.

Thus, an approach evolves which seems logical to us when faced with an acutely or chronically infected person: the prescription of an initial treatment based on the clinical indications revealed on first examining the patient and on the knowledge of any previous history, such as related factors. This treatment should be started as soon as the sample has been taken, even if it means adjusting it on completion of the aromatogramme.

Finally, the study of aromatogrammes brings out another important factor in favour of natural therapeutics as opposed to conventional antibiotics: the question of *resistance*. Indeed, quite apart from the abusive use of antibiotics, the dramatic increase recently in the polymorphous resistance of germs to all types of antibiotic, sometimes even the latest ones, is well known. So, the repeated study of aromatogrammes during the recurring evolution of former chronic infections, the eradication of which cannot take place overnight, has enabled us to establish that in fact there was very little resistance to the oils and that more often than not, give or take a little, we were finding that the effects of the same oils remained almost unchanged.

This can be very easily explained because we have already said that, in the same way that plants act on the soil, oils determined by the aromatogramme have their greatest effect on the area of the body which is most likely to favour the development of germs. *Phyto-aromatherapy* acts on this area and, moreover, we often include similarly active catalysers.

In the course of time, certain aspects of the ailment disappear although their elimination is insufficient to destroy all the germs. Then one simply has to adjust the treatment to suit the new conditions.

4.   Some Drawbacks of Modern Medication

What can be said to constitute safe and healthy treatment? I would offer this definition: any substance or process which is non-toxic and constant in its effects when faced with the same symptoms. So, to take a simple example, natural sleep remains the real treatment for a state of fatigue brought about by staying awake too long. The effect of hydrotherapy does not change with the passing of time, nor does the effect of balneotherapy whether taken by itself or in association with plants and essences such as heather, lavender, thyme, rosemary, lime and seaweed. The effect on two similar conditions will be the same as it has always been throughout the centuries such treatment has been given. The organism cannot become "habituated" in the pejorative sense of the word – i.e. no longer able to derive any benefit – any more than it can become habituated to leavened bread, pure olive or sunflower oil, organically grown vegetables, pure mountain air or personal hygiene. The results remain the same; they do not lessen over any length of time.

On the other hand, the organism does become habituated to chemically synthesised narcotics, and the result is known as *tolerance*. One may start out by taking a single sleeping-pill at supper or a suppository at bed-time; before long one may well have reached the stage of taking anything from four to ten pills and two or three suppositories and still be unable to get to sleep. And so one changes the make of pill – and fashion usually dictates the choice. One chooses the latest product on the market, and the process begins all over again.

An old ship-owner, weighed down with domestic and financial problems, drugged himself like this for thirty years until, weary of his failure to enjoy a proper night's sleep in spite of the latest discoveries in supersoporifics, he took to heart the humble advice of a country woman. An infusion of a mixture of orange flowers and leaves gave him back the gift of sleep in a single week.

Accustomed to reacting to the different things that attack it, the body will become habituated to everything which is in any way adulterated, harmful or toxic, by a kind of mithridatising process.[1] Every case of intoxication, however insignificant, brings with it some damage to the body; though when the effects of the drug begin to wear off, the body becomes able to fight back again and sooner or later will take the upper

1   Mithridatism – tolerance to certain toxic substances acquired by ingesting progressively larger doses of a given poison.

hand to escape from the influence of the chemical product. But once its capacity for defence is exhausted, the body soon becomes prey to a variety of mishaps. Marcel Perrault observed that "there is too much dangerous medication and it is often unnecessary to prescribe it. Some times it is best to return to a state of total medicinal peace".

One can become habituated to anything – even aspirin, except when it is found to provoke bleeding of the stomach or a blood condition. Tolerance to aspirin has reached such a level that one can point to a kind of aspirin-taking mania – "aspirinitis" someone has called it. In the United States a population of 220,000,000 people consumes 42,000,000 tablets every day – that is to say an average of 100 tablets per adult per year. This excessive use is no doubt put down to the prevalence of migraines whether of hepatic or menstrual or any other origin, the proliferation of various kinds of neuralgia, a way of life which entails too high a degree of excitement and generates anxieties, and other conditions as well. But it is also true that the aspirin's effectiveness was originally considered in terms of a single tablet, and that now three times or ten times the dose – or even half a bottle – seems to be needed for it to have any effect. Several of my own patients over a two-year period have absorbed between 3,000 and 6,000 tablets of various kinds.[2]

Faced with this vast consumer market, the drug manufacturers base their tactics on originality and so they produce their tablets in a bewildering variety of shapes and sizes – square ones, diamond-shaped ones, even animal-shaped ones for children.

The tolerance caused by antibiotics has a relatively long history. Let me give you some practical results of antibiotic treatment from first-hand experience. During the winter of 1944–45 when I was Medical Officer to a company of the *Corps France*, I injected – as did every army doctor at the time – all seriously wounded patients with 25,000 units of penicillin every three hours until they could be evacuated. This method paved the way for countless successes in the subsequent treatment of the wounds. Many a soldier owed a limb, even life, to the existence of this precious antibiotic. Then, when I was attached to the Surgical Faculty of the Hospital of Evacuation 412 at Besançon in February 1945, I had an opportunity of studying the spectacular effects of penicillin in the treat-

---

2 The French in no way lag behind in this matter, consuming 400 tons of medicaments, or 3.6 kilos per person, per year – and this includes 4 billion aspirin tablets. It is true that, as the Americans have pointed out, "medicines in France are the cheapest in the world"; in fact one American pharmaceutical bulletin, *The Better Life*, has produced the following table to show the hours of work required in five representative industrial countries to pay for the same brand of tranquilliser (this is presumably based on the average wage of a manual worker):

In France	1 hour 57 minutes
In Italy	4 hours 46 minutes
In Germany	3 hours 18 minutes
In Japan	7 hours 38 minutes
In U.S.A.	2 hours 18 minutes

ment of even very severe war wounds. One evening, after the battle of Colmar, we received more than 400 wounded soldiers in the space of a few hours; I had to go to Strasbourg to pick up the penicillin we would need. It was a real expedition of a journey then, at night, in February '45, and the black ice and shell craters on the road and the worn-out shock absorbers of a jeep which under normal circumstances would have been pensioned off long since, combined to mount an unremitting attack on both my concentration and my spine. After travelling all night I came into the penicillin depot in Strasbourg at around 5 in the morning. As day was breaking, two 50-bottle boxes were handed over to me, and I saw them safely back to Hospital 412. Each of these bottles contained 100,000 units of penicillin, and with 100 bottles we had altogether 10 million units of the antibiotic – enough in those days to save about 60 legs (between 100,000 and 200,000 units were then found to be sufficient) or, as we put it, 20 "stomachs" or as many "chests".

What an anachronism these figures are! In order to reach a useful therapeutic dose today one has to inject a patient with several million units daily over a period of from three to upwards of twenty days – and this would be for a feverish condition, straightforward bronchitis or simple nasal catarrh. The essences of eucalyptus, cinnamon, cloves, pine needles, turpentine, thyme or niaouli would have dealt with such conditions in a matter of 24 to 48 hours – eight days at the most for the stubborn cases.

If we turn to accident or post-operative cases, we find the almost universal automatic reaction is to administer systematically several million units of penicillin a day, more often than not in association with streptomycin, terramycin or any one of a number of other antibiotics, according to the surgeon's particular beliefs. "Penicillin may be injected without risk for weeks or months on end in massive doses of 80 to 100 million units a day," wrote G. Bickel; but an American doctor has demanded that these illogical and pernicious practices be banned.[3]

The sulphonamide drugs, which preceded antibiotics and were thought in their day to be the panacea sought after down the centuries, have suffered exactly the same fate.

One example should be enough. When in 1941–42 I was working as medical assistant to Professor Maurice Favre, head of the Department of Dermato-Venerology at the Hospital Grange Blanche in Lyons, I had the opportunity to study the curative effects of a new sulphonamide in the treatment of blennorrhagia. Two tablets of this medication given every two hours would at that time cause the disappearance of the gonococcus from urethral secretions in 14 to 16 hours. A maximum of 16 tablets of 0.5g each was sufficient to deal with scalding urine. The results were of course always confirmed by microscopic examination. At the same time,

---

3   Meyers of Chicago has calculated that post-operative infection has been present in 1.3% of his patients not treated with antibiotics, and in 4% of those undergoing routine antibiotic treatment.

this discovery had taken the wind out of the sails of a host of braggarts who had made much of their "woman's diseases".

But the news soon spread and the treatment became debased, for by putting their whole trust in the extraordinary properties of this new substance, the entire specialist community absorbed two or three tablets a day in the hope of becoming immune to the microbe and therefore more certain of attracting customers. It was the gonococcus that was immunised. The original 14–16 tablets soon became 40, then 80, until in the end they ceased to have any reliable effect, so that there was a great sigh of relief when penicillin appeared and once more we thought that we were out of the wood, that this time we had banished venereal disease from our anxiety list for good. But the antibiotics in their turn lost their power against these infections, whose agents – the habit having stuck – immunised themselves; and this is why within the last few years venereal diseases, which for more than 20 years were thought to have disappeared, have been making a comeback into the ranks of risks to be feared and avoided.

Yet, as with so many other conditions, the answer to these illnesses might well be found in the use of plants and essences, many of which have been known for a long time. Deterpenated essence of lavender taken in pearls of .05 to .1g at a dosage of between 2 and 10 pearls a day is far and away the most effective against gonorrhoea, though the essences of sandalwood, cedarwood and copaiba are effective enough, likewise the essences of juniper, the rhizome of couch grass, the buds of the umbrella-fir, garlic and others. Syphilitic sores and chancres are cured by the application of deterpenated essence of lavender, and sassafras makes an excellent additional treatment for syphilis.

The arrival of synthetic substances has quite wrongly made people forget these medicaments or regard them with scorn. A detailed study would soon show which essences are most active in the treatment of gonorrhoea and other venereal diseases, and what dosage would be required.

When I served as surgeon in the Advanced Surgical Unit Number 1 in Tonkin from 1950 to 1952, and later in the Evacuation Hospital 415 in Saigon, I had the time and opportunity to study the relative effectiveness of sulphonamides and antibiotics on people of different races. I was able to establish the effect of these medicines to be much more pronounced in Vietnamese or African patients than their European counterparts, for these nationalities had for the most part, never been treated in this way before; one could therefore predict quite marked differences in their method of action.

I could give numerous examples here of the current impotence of numerous once highly effective synthetic and antibiotic medications against a wide range of conditions. In the long run, for all the spectacular results they had at first, they have not justified their reputations. If there were not, still, a slight aura of mystery surrounding this area, it would be perfectly obvious that we are coming up against growing numbers of conditions which have become resistant to the treatments that formerly cured them. Generally speaking, this phenomenon is a result of the indiscriminate use of the medications, often in defiance of informed medical opinion, by the patients themselves. But I have a further point: increasingly, their indiscriminate use can be seen to be potentially dangerous. The very fact that, out of several hundred bactericidal or bacteriostatic substances isolated or synthesised in the laboratory, only 20 or so will have a therapeutic use is surely a clear demonstration that in the main they are far from inoffensive. Even those antibiotics sanctioned by wide and constant use are not without toxicity; if penicillin is not strictly toxic it is nevertheless responsible for a large number of allergic reactions.

Antibiotics can set off allergies, and this happens most frequently in countries where they are in general use. The widespread diffusion of penicillin, its systematic and at times indiscriminate use in mild infections, together with its abuse in such pharmaceutical preparations as toothpaste, can explain the steadily increasing numbers of people in the West who have become sensitised to it. Antibiotics can also have detrimental side-effects on the blood, from slight anaemia or a simple fall in the number of white corpuscles ("of little import") to the total disappearance of the white cells. According to Bickel, streptomycin has proved to be the most hostile towards the formation of blood corpuscles. Again, there is a danger of *toxic effects*; the most regrettable problems attributable to streptomycin are those affecting the nervous system and, in particular, hearing and the sense of balance. I have also witnessed the onset of lethargy, difficulty in breathing and even cases of total deafness affecting both ears. The region of the ear is susceptible to toxic effects of other antibiotics too. I think it must serve the real interests of these medicines as well as those of the patient who may benefit from them without any unfortunate complications to describe their possible side-effects in certain circumstances. It is surely more than reasonable to refrain from rushing blindly into new modes of therapy which have not had time to prove their worth. As Professor Marcel Perrault wrote "It is often a virtue to be conservative in medical matters."

Again, antibiotics have been found to possess *renal toxicity*; some also can cause *nervous complications*, real psychic disturbances, violent attacks comparable with epileptic fits. Cases of *secondary infection*[4] may occasionally be observed, and aureomycin, and penicillin and streptomycin in association, are often responsible for the appearance of stubborn entero-colitis (de Vernejoul, Cook). The destruction of the normal intestinal flora[5] by these medications, and the consequent proliferation of staphylococcus may lead to death which may come about in a "terrifying

4   A new infection contracted by a patient already infected and not yet cured.

5   The microbial flora which is indispensable to health is destroyed along with the germs of the infection which led to the use of antibiotics in the first place. Many present-day intestinal troubles may analogously be attributed to food with chemical additives.

fashion". This kind of complication is most often found when antibiotics have been administered either before or after surgery on the stomach or intestine, and a growing number of surgeons are speaking out against systematic injections of antibiotics for operations of this nature.

To sum up: if penicillin is most often responsible for allergic complications, chloramphenicol for conditions of the blood, tetracyclines for entero-colitis and so on, we may be justified in supposing *all antibiotics capable of giving rise to further diseases. This is a risk one cannot ignore.* The above facts were confirmed by a study of the records of the US Ministry of Health (1953–1957). As far as *toxic side-effects* are concerned, "one can no longer speak of risk but of semi-certitude, for a sufficient dose will always provoke the same phenomena". One might therefore think it an adequate precaution to keep the dosage below this level, yet it has been proved – in the cases of numerous medications and chemical products introduced into food substances – that even though small doses in themselves appear to entail no unfortunate effects, their accumulation in the organism by repeated consumption may, in the long run, lead to degenerative diseases, in particular cancer (Professors Redding and Truhaut). These problems with their tragic consequences are the current preoccupation of many doctors throughout the world.

"Antibiotics should not be used except in cases of absolute necessity" was the conclusion of the International Congress of Chemotherapy held in Naples in 1961. Authors of numerous papers were in agreement that antibiotics were not the ideal solution to the problem of reinforcing the body's natural defence mechanisms. Again and again the severely toxic effects that antibiotics are capable of causing were underlined, likewise the dangers of tolerance. Of course it should be stressed that there is no question here of ignoring the brilliant possibilities they offer in certain very serious conditions (tubercular meningitis, for instance, whose treatment has been revolutionised by antibiotics). But if it is logical, and in truth essential, to take the risks inherent in their use when the severity of the condition justifies it, the disadvantages of these medicaments must surely forbid their being administered systematically or lightly for illnesses susceptible enough to less dangerous treatments. A serious condition obviously authorises the use of antibiotics, and in high doses; but one should be aware that "the price of a cure may be a permanent disability".

Nor are the sulphonamides innocent of side-effects, and serious ones at that. Their spectacular success quickly multiplied their general use, and it is not surprising that numerous complications made themselves apparent – which is, incidentally, one of the reasons why these medicaments were so readily eclipsed by the arrival of penicillin when its harmful effects were still unknown. Complications involving kidney damage are commonest as a result of sulphonamide treatment, together with the reactions of sensitisation, i.e. fever on the ninth day and skin eruptions – not generally worrying, but the possible precursors of more serious reactions such as nephritis, problems affecting the blood or hepatitis, the blood conditions being either benign and transitory or, as in the case of antibiotics, capable of leading to death. These major problems constitute the ultimate risk taken every time a sulpha drug is given; even the most recent of these drugs, administered in doses four to six times lower than in the past, are as potentially dangerous. (Sulphonamide complications have been specially studied by Salvaggio and Gonzales, Tisdale, Holsinger and Welch).

Sulphonamides and antibiotics are not the only medicaments capable of causing tolerance or producing organic disorders. Statistics used by the Registrar-General for England and Wales show that, in the period 1957–58, 265 deaths were due to therapeutic reactions and these included 39 as a result of radiation, 20 deaths following blood transfusions and 11 after anti-convulsant treatment. As far as medicaments were concerned, 13 deaths were caused by the use of chloramphenicol, 11 followed the use of chlorpromazine, 9 deaths resulted from anticoagulant treatment, 5 from the use of phenylbutazone, 4 from gold and 16 from insulin, 14 of which were by hypoglycemic coma, 10 from sulpha drugs and 8 from penicillin, the rest being caused variously by the use of corticosteroids, anti-thyroid drugs, preparations with an iron base, cytotoxic drugs, mercurial diuretics and aspirin (British Medical Journal, 1960).

Therapeutic accidents are clearly the order of the day. The steadily growing number of published articles shows that in the final analysis every chemical and synthetic therapy contains an element of risk, the most anodyne as well as the most violent, the commonest as well as the very latest thing. Professor Conté predicted it in his inaugural lecture of 1961, when he said, "after arteriosclerosis, cancer and road accidents, *therapeutic illnesses* will one day overtake tuberculosis and syphilis, those rightful terrors of our parents, in the list of 'parasites on society'." This is now confirmed to be true. Ignorance of the dangers certainly allowed the early experimenters to be daring. Certainly there are times when boldness is needed and when to save a patient condemned to certain death medicine must take a chance on the unknown. But in daily practice the general practitioner, and still more the increasing numbers of patients who think they can look after themselves, should be fully aware of the possibility of therapeutic risk.

To play my part in disseminating this vital knowledge, I shall continue with instances of specific damage. Phenylbutazone and its derivatives can provoke allergic reactions of the skin and agranulocytosis (disappearance of the white corpuscles); cases of mortality have been published (Gsell, von Rechenberg). There have also been cases of gastrointestinal bleeding – haemorrhagic gastritis, with eventual ulceration, may in fact be provoked by phenylbutazone even when it is injected, and for this reason the treatment is forbidden to all patients with gastric ulcers or with no more than a history of digestive troubles. Salts of gold are responsible for a number of skin lesions, and lesions of the mucus membrane. They are known to have caused blood conditions, some of them serious, also serious kidney conditions and polyneuritis. Synthetic drugs supposed to prevent or cure malaria are always more or less harmful to man, causing skin troubles, anaemia, eyesight problems and such psychic problems as excitement, hallucination and delirium.

Several authors have reported on the serious condition which certain viral infections, may conceal in subjects who have taken corticosteroids over a long period. In *Vaccins et Serums*,[6] Professor Pierre Chassange sums up three main areas of danger inherent in cortisone treatment:

"The first point is that cortisone derivatives certainly reduce the resistance of the organism to agents of infection; this has been proved both experimentally and clinically. An experimental example may be found in the sensitisation of animals in the laboratory to the poliomyelitis virus following cortisone treatment; as a clinical example, on the other hand, everyone knows that certain viral diseases such as chicken-pox may be aggravated as a result of prolonged cortisone treatment prior to the infection.

"Second is the influence exerted by cortisone derivatives on the process of immunisation, in particular the immunisation process acquired during the course of an illness or after the injection of a vaccine. Prolonged cortisone treatment hinders the establishment of immunity, and even if it is short it has an adverse effect.

"The third point – a strictly practical one – is that cortisone treatment should never be given without simultaneous active treatment against infection, and by that I mean verified treatment against infection; for if cortisone treatment is associated with the administering of some antibiotic to which the germ is not susceptible, one risks the most serious consequences."

Cortisone and its numerous derivatives can cause complications in patients with recto-colitis, and often bring about a profound alteration of the intestinal wall. In the treatment of rheumatism, cortisone has only a suspensive effect masking the symptoms without altering their development (9 cases improved out of 546 treated – Bauer and Ragan). Treatment using cortisone or analogous drugs can cause the perforation of a gastric ulcer, give an impetus to unrecognised tuberculosis and lead to psychic problems. Surely we are dealing here with a method of treatment which in the majority of cases it would be better to do without. At the very least there should be a clamp-down on patients who play around dangerously with these substances themselves, swallowing them with as much thought as if they were eating sweets. Methods of prescription ought to be laid down by the doctor alone; only he has the knowledge to be able to judge the situation properly and act responsibly.

6   Doin, édit, 1961.

As to vaccination, I have no desire to stir up in this book a debate of long-standing which probably has a good deal of life in it yet. Systematic vaccination is not always harmless, but doctors are aware of this and should note any counter-indications. In 1957 Professors Delore and Charpy called attention to several serious cases of reactivation of tuberculosis following revaccination for smallpox.[7] It should also be noted that smallpox revaccination can produce an infarct about nine days after scarification, As early as 1955, in *Archives des Maladies du coeur* Mathieu was recommending that vaccination should be avoided by elderly people with coronary conditions.

In 1959, Dr Delagrange, house physician at the Hopitaux de Paris, gave his opinion on various repercussions of vaccination in the *Cahiers Laënnec*. He wrote: "A deep-seated pre-existing complaint may be aggravated by vaccination. . . . There are, of course, certain cases (they are very rare) of nephropathy (kidney-disease) following vaccination in healthy people, but it should not be forgotten that this nephritis may be due to the reawakening of old or cured nephropathy. It is equally difficult to judge cases of the reawakening of old or stablised tuberculosis.

"In these contentious cases one should always ask whether the shock of vaccine on a latent germ may give rise to a disease at that particular moment. Certain observations do not exclude the possibility that the vaccine modifies the virus allowing it to provoke a real illness, or that it sensitises the subject, making him less resistant to the virus."

In 1963, during a discussion on *the mechanism of immunity to infection*, Dr Jonas Salk suggested that it was unnecessary to vaccinate an entire population to eliminate a viral disease. The disappearance of smallpox from certain areas of the world was manifest proof of less than total immunisation. It was difficult to cast doubt on the completeness of its disappearance, bearing in mind how long a period had passed without a single case of smallpox being recorded. The absence of the disease in those countries was not necessarily due to the perseverance of the agents of vaccination; indeed, in some of them vaccination was no longer carried out systematically. Nor was the extinction of smallpox due to the solid individual immunity of people not yet vaccinated, as was shown by cases of imported smallpox. Thus we were presented with the practical possibility of obtaining the worldwide extinction of smallpox by means of a properly designed programme of immunisation which need not require either the vaccination of every single person or continuous revaccination, The same "immunological mechanism" which had partially eliminated smallpox could also eliminate poliomyelitis and other viral diseases (VIII International Congress of Microbiology. Pittsburgh, USA).

The principle of the "immunological mechanism" put forward by Dr

---

7   Note that in England, the US and Canada, smallpox vaccination is no longer obligatory.

Salk seems to me both valid and worthy of support; I have for a long time believed it to be a combination of cosmic factors and the modification imposed on them by "civilisation", and have no doubt that in this conjunction, vaccination does not always play the capital role with which it is credited today.

Turning to the use of "tranquillisers", "anti-depressants" and numerous appetite-reducing pills, there has been ample opportunity for the public to read about the appalling results made apparent in the birth of deformed babies. "Cases of congenital malformation have increased with the use of 'tranquillisers'," Professor Giroud deposed before the French Academy of Medicine in 1962. "We have ourselves produced experimental evidence of the effects of thalidomide[8] in these cases of malformation. But is it the only substance responsible?" For the incidence of congenital malformation seemed to have increased in the last few years, even in France where thalidomide had not been marketed commercially, as a result of the use of other "tranquillisers". Professor Giroud advised that the administering of drugs to pregnant women ought to be kept to the absolute minimum, above all during the first month of gestation, "using, where possible, *ancient remedies* which have already proved that they are harmless". It is among those natural aromatic plants and essences which have been used for centuries as sedatives, tonics and regulators of the appetite that the desired "ancient remedies" will most easily be found.

Apart from the terrible result of permanent damage to a foetus, certain synthetic drugs can often be held responsible for other side-effects. They are the more often put to use because they "respond to a particular need of our age, and because a large number of these substances are regularly used therapeutically". They are a danger to the public, which tends to take them indiscriminately as a panacea. Furthermore, classifying them is difficult and the terms "tranquilliser", "nerve sedative", "neuro-plegic", "mood-elevator" and "ataractic" are often used in a very imprecise manner.

All doctors may observe the same problems and disasters which these particular products cause: jactitation, for instance, or obnubilation; trembling reminiscent of Parkinson's disease; various conditions of the "neuro-vegetative" series, including vertigo, palpitations, spasms; "paradoxical" reactions, with excitation similar to delirium following the administration of sedatives, also increased depression when so-called tonics are used. It is not uncommon to witness reactions which exceed the desired goal and threaten to transform a state of mania into anxiety, or a depressive state into excitation. Finally, it should never be forgotten

---

8 Dr Torsten Hafstroem, Chief Medical Officer of the Southern Hospital, Stockholm, believes that thalidomide can cause problems in adults, particularly circulation problems and neuroses.

that all these drugs considerably increase the damage alcohol causes; this property, which is insufficiently recognised, may well be one of the root causes of severe accidents on the road or in the factory. Apart from all these drawbacks, one ought also to note the frequency of allergic skin reactions which may even affect the person looking after the patient, causing a kind of eczema as a result of contact. There have been cases of jaundice which can lead to fatty degeneration of the heart. These side-effects, which sometimes prove fatal, are caused by an immoderate use of anti-depressant drugs. In America they have given rise to a genuine panic (S. A. Sandler) whose reverberations I certainly felt when I travelled there in 1970.

We should take note too of fatal accidents whose cause is not always explained, of pains in muscles and joints, and various – some serious – reactions of the blood, etc. Moreover, Dr John Michael has spoken out against the excessive and prolonged use of anti-coagulants in the treatment of myocardial infarction. The study of 5,000 cases treated prophylactically and over a long period with anti-coagulants shows no greater a survival rate than among patients receiving no anti-coagulant treatment. The mortality rate among 446 patients who had recently suffered myocardial infarction and had undergone anti-coagulant treatment and a similar group who had not been so treated was calculated to be 34% in either case.

The doubtful benefits of this treatment should therefore be weighed against the risk – and it is a serious one – of haemorrhage. Dr Michael refers to a 3–4% death rate in the study. Furthermore, anti-coagulants have no positive effect on the diminution of the calibre of the artery, but interrupting the treatment once it has begun predisposes the patient to thrombosis and even arterial occlusion. Other serious side-effects that should be mentioned include intestinal occlusion, spitting of blood, cerebral haemorrhage, cutaneous necrosis and pericardial and genital outpourings of blood. *Even if experiment continues, this routine use of anti-coagulants must stop. The author demands that patients should not be subjected to this inefficient and dangerous treatment.* He asks that new and original research be undertaken to try and understand the mechanism of atherosclerosis, and the reasons for the frequency of certain of its localisations, for as far as he is concerned, the risk of haemorrhage is not counter-balanced by the doubtful effects of a reduction of coagulability (Annual Congress of the British Medical Association, London).

Plants and aromatic essences together with a natural diet have always done and will continue to do better than the habitual prescription of anti-coagulants.

Reading more or less at random in medical journals I discovered another example of the dangers of chemo-therapy. The nasal inhalation of certain vaso-constrictory products (i.e. products with the property of contracting blood vessels or capillaries) was contra-indicated for the baby at the breast; their use had been linked with cases of prostration, pallor, chilling and nasal obstruction by secondary infiltration from the original action of the medicament. Again, a shampoo containing selenium, generally prescribed for loss of hair, has in several cases produced more or less total baldness.

"Chemists," wrote Professor Delbet,[9] "with prodigious and enlightened skill juggle with atoms, radicals and molecules, producing new substances each more active than the last. . . . All these substances are *toxic* to the organism."

I shall conclude this account by examining briefly some general considerations relating to aspirin, in the light of a recent study. This study clearly shows how vital it is to be extremely cautious in the distribution of chemical drugs – even those which appear most innocuous.

"Aspirin is found in use everywhere. Its remarkable effectiveness against ills of all descriptions has made it a product which is used every day; it is beyond medical prescription or monitoring, but its harmlessness seemed to have been empirically demonstrated and an established fact. However, since 1938, this familiar drug has seen its innocence questioned in the very country which had adopted it as a kind of symbol of domestic health. In England it has been observed that severe stomach bleeding followed the absorption of normal doses of aspirin, and it was established that in patients suffering from ulcers it played an important role in aggravating the symptoms: at the very least it encouraged gastric haemorrhage in one case out of eight. By systematic testing of the blood in the stools of hospitalised rheumatic patients with no past history of gastric trouble who were being treated with aspirin in daily doses of 0.75 to 3g, Stubbe revealed the existence of haemorrhaging of unknown origin in 70%. The toxicity of the aspirin may also make itself apparent in the liver and nervous system, especially in the case of children. An overdose, whether accidental or intentional (this method of suicide seems particularly favoured in Anglo-Saxon countries), may provoke convulsive crises and lead to death."[10]

Allergic reactions to aspirin, such as urticaria, Quincke's oedema (infiltration of the face and larynx), spasmodic coryza and bronchial asthma, are not uncommon. In a published series of eleven observations on asthmatic subjects, Blamoutier includes two cases of death which rapidly followed a single, weak dose of aspirin. "The medical practitioner must therefore be extremely cautious with patients possessing this sensitisation. He must ensure that the medicines he prescribes contain no aspirin and must draw the patient's attention to the danger this kind of medicament possesses for him."

During the study day devoted to the life and destiny of man in our civilisation which was held in Paris in 1962, John Rostand I understand was outspoken against the triple dangers of radio-activity, X-rays – and the abusive use of medicines. I also understand that Cunnot, confining

9 *Politique Préventive de Cancer* (Denoël, édit, 1944).

10 See Appendices II

himself to a limited aspect of the problem, declared that "the influx of new and effective medicines for the treatment of tuberculosis should not make us forget the ancient treatment using creosote derived from beech-wood – indeed, they should contribute to its rehabilitation." With the creosote of course, as with other medications derived from vegetable substances, there is no risk. Or again, consider the drug "MER 29", long regarded as effective against cholesterol: it had to be withdrawn from the market, first in the US and then in other countries, on account of its various side-effects – baldness, loss of body hair, cataracts and skin troubles.

A substance of American origin, WIN 18446, first used in the treatment of dysentery, has also shown itself capable of putting a temporary stop to the production of sperm. A dose of 1 gram a day has this effect for as long as it is taken, until 100 days after the treatment is finished when fertility is restored. J. McLoud of Cornell University is confident that this should prove a sound weapon in the fight to cut the birth-rate, arguing that it is both cheap and safe (Drugs and Cosm. Ind., May 1961). The reader must draw his own conclusion, for "safe" seems at the least to be a premature claim.

Inquiries are now being held in several countries into the ramifications of the drugs I have been discussing. In some countries, notably Belgium, Sweden, Denmark, Great Britain, Canada, Italy, Holland and the United States, various measures have been taken to restrict the sale of drugs and this applies in particular to neuroleptics (sedatives), sea-sickness pills, obesity pills and even medicines containing bismuth salts and quinine. Some of these substances have been temporarily withdrawn from the pharmaceutical market, and others which had previously been on open sale may now only be obtained with a medical prescription. In 1962, a declaration of intent was made by the French Ministry of Public Health to create "a national committee to co-ordinate research into the terato-genic effects of drugs", i.e. effects which produce monsters.

As early as 1960, Brun, Kalb and Possetto were writing as follows in the *Presse Médicale*:

"In the last fifteen years the number of drugs has multiplied at a bewildering rate, and it has become difficult to see one's way clearly through the modern pharmacopoeia. Overwhelmed by powerful publicity which substitutes unthinking and automatic action for sound medically-based diagnosis, doctors nowadays take the risk of satisfying what is a real hunger for drugs, a hunger well-known to their patients. Today everything has to be done quickly; one must act 'energetically'. If results are slow in coming, the drug must be changed, several times a week if necessary, lest the patient change his doctor. New prescriptions are added to old in such a way that finally drops, tablets, suppositories and injections multiply and mingle in a hectic whirl which often threatens to make the situation worse and discredit the diagnosis.

"Whether to do too much or not to do enough is a recurrent dilemma, especially when it is not very clear what ought to be done.

"From another point of view, the patients have also changed – one is perhaps too ready to forget this. For first of all there are certain patients who have acquired hypersensitivity and powerful defence reactions sometimes more terrible than the original aggression itself. Woe betide the person who, confronted with such cases, ventures to bring back various old-fashioned remedies which cured the whole whilst destroying very little – the days of brandy and syrup of buckthorn are by and large over!

"Furthermore – and this second point is most important – the abundance and repetition of administered drugs, particularly antibiotics, together with the abuse of stimulants means that more and more often patients are in a highly complex state of sensitivity which peculiarly modifies their individual reactions to therapies which might otherwise be considered innocuous.

"We seem to be reaching a dangerous stage. The considerable benefit which the discovery of new drugs has brought with it has allowed the removal of a number of processes weakened by conditioned defence reflexes against therapies which the body will now come to regard as aggressors.

"We are not talking here about complications with tragic associations, nor of accidental overdoses which may easily be detected or corrected. What does concern us are the misleading manifestations which more often than not are signs of the body's sensitisation or saturation during both acute and chronic conditions, and in respect of valid and normal doses of a given drug. The disappearance of these misleading symptoms is conditioned by therapeutic peace – that is to say, the total suppression over a certain period of all aggressive reaction to drugs of whatever sort.

"More often than not this seems to us to explain the constant success of certain drugs which, administered in minute doses, give peace both to the body and to the mind; for in the final analysis nothing is more important than to appear to give everything when in fact you are giving nothing at all."

In fact, as Chassangene and Georges-Fanet emphasised elsewhere,[11] there is often considerable danger in prescribing hormone treatments which are "almost always useless anyway" for children. The virilising effects of these drugs in girls are well-known, but much less is known about those hormones "whose use entails so many disasters: ovaries which develop tumours" for instance. Naturally, these hormones are indicated in just a few cases for grown women, and have just as many disadvantages as for children. Furthermore, when a woman is pregnant these hormones are capable – as has been shown in experiments with animals – of producing a bisexual state in the child by virilising a foetus which was originally female.

11 P. Chassangene and L. Georges-Fanet: *Quelques thérapeutiques dangereuses chez l'enfant.*

"The doctor in his capacity as clinician should mistrust every automatic reaction, and think of the individual for whom he is caring at that moment – an individual who may be hypersensitive, exhausted or saturated by a succession or accumulation of drugs and whose toxic aggression may be worse than the illness.

"In many cases we should return to the modest attitudes which doctors had in the past. They knew that each organism reacts and is cured in its own way and in its own time, and that provided the confidence of the patient is aroused and maintained the moment of cure will surely come." These words of M. Perrault remind us of the old saying, "It is better to look after one's health than one's illness" or, as it was put hundreds of years ago, "The best medicine is to have no need of medicine".

5.   A Multitude of Uses

Besides their antiseptic and bactericidal properties, many essences have *antiviral* properties. I do not know if a systematic study has been undertaken to determine this action in relation to different essential oils, but a mixture of essences has in my own experience had remarkable success in numerous cases of *shingles*.

This condition, caused by a filterable virus,[1] is generally painful and begins with violent attacks of neuralgia, often localised on the left or right side of the thorax, or equally on the left or right hemi-face (ophthalmic shingles, which may lead to the loss of an eye), sometimes extending to the arm. It is characterised by an eruption of vesicles reminiscent of herpes arranged in groups along the path of the sensitive nerves of the skin, always on one side of the body only. Normally accompanied by severe pain, they evolve into ulcers. The elective localisation of shingles on the nervous system has caused the condition to be called "posterior poliomyelitis". It can develop in a very serious manner, the ulceration leading to extensive sores which are painful and tenacious. I know of a doctor's wife who had sores on the thorax lasting several months, and her life during this period was sheer hell. The pain may even persist for months or years after the apparent end of the disease; there have been victims who have suffered from three to fourteen years after the disappearance of the vesicles.

At the moment there is no specific treatment for shingles and it is still often treated with soothing ointments and, not very convincingly, the ingestion of vitamins and the use of X-rays. But the mixture of essential oils can suppress shingles in a *maximum* of one week if the condition is treated during the first days of its appearance (a little more time is required if the condition has already developed).

A patient came to see me one day, desperate about the prospect of cancelling a business trip abroad because of shingles which had appeared three days earlier. He was due to depart in one week's time. I got him to agree to make no change in his plans: twice-daily applications of

1   The term *filterable virus* is given to numerous germs specific to particular diseases (e.g. poliomyelitis, aphthous fever, smallpox, influenza), represented by particles so small that they are able to pass through the normal filters used to retain microbes. The filterable viruses are invisible to the ordinary microscope, but their image has been established thanks to the electron microscope.

aromatic essences and a daily intra-muscular injection of citral (a constituent of some essential oils) cleared up the condition in three days.

Influenza, too, is caused by a filterable virus, which by itself gives rise to a harmless cold but in association with various microbes may lead to broncho-pulmonary conditions of varying degrees of seriousness according to the patient and the epidemic. It is a well-known fact that every year "flu" is responsible for several thousand deaths.

Many essences (e.g. cinnamon, pine needles, thyme, lemon) have marked effects on this condition, and patients treated with these essences for a variety of complaints seem to get through the winter without trouble.[2]

The antiseptic power of these essences is complemented by their cicatrising properties. Found chiefly among the Labiatae (e.g. lavender, sage, thyme, rosemary), these properties can assist in the healing of abrasions or infected wounds, leg ulcers and fistulas. I can cite the case of a young man who had had a fistula near the base of his spine for many years; yet the flow was stopped in a matter of days with a mixture of essences of lavender, thyme and pine needles. Another case concerned a seriously ill patient who for several months had had an artificial anus on the left side as a result of cancer of the large intestine; this incision had become granulated, swollen, very inflamed and painful. Treated with a mixture of essential oils in diluted form on compresses twice a day, the incision took on a much healthier aspect and the inflammation was completely checked within a week.

This case demonstrates that *cancerous wounds* are amenable to treatment with aromatic essences. The essences have this healing effect because of their ability to increase the blood supply to the tissues, and this assists both the detergent action of the white corpuscles and cell regeneration. Aromatic wines, which were so prevalent at the time of the Renaissance, had an excellent reputation in this respect and numerous writings stressed their value in the treatment of burns, abrasions and infected wounds. *Gangrenous wounds* may also be treated successfully with essential oils. Acting as powerful disinfectants, they bring about a true embalming process which leads to cicatrisation.

R. M. Gattefossé has published a relevant personal case history. He suffered serious burns to the hands in a laboratory explosion, and the wounds soon became gangrenous; he was able to effect a perfect cure using essence of lavender. I myself made use of the healing properties of essences in wartime surgery on some of my patients in Tonkin, and though having only a very limited quantity of my own aromatic essences I was unable to treat as many patients as I should have liked, the results that I did obtain were consistent.

During the 1914–18 war, applications of aromatic essences were common in a variety of civilian and military hospitals. In 1915,

2　In 1972 a number of scientific communications claimed that antibiotics were ineffectual against influenza.

Mencière was using various compositions of essential oils in predetermined doses, for their bactericidal and healing properties. He used a water emulsion for wet dressings and solutions of ether, at 10g per thousand, for large wounds where a considerable amount of tissue had been lost; he also used dressings with aromatic ointments. In 1917, Duchesne perfected a formula with a base of vaseline and ether, which contained camphor, gomenol and balsam of Peru.

Where aromatic essences are used, healing takes place quickly without dangerous toxicity or the formation of scars. Some essential oils in fact have quite startling effects on old, keloid or unsightly scars. I can instance one patient, an attractive young woman, who had been burnt in childhood by a poultice applied to her neck and the upper part of her chest while it was too hot, leaving an ugly scar. In three months, compresses soaked in diluted essences and applied twice daily caused a considerable reduction of the marks. It is a matter of genuine regret that these methods are not more widely used; their reintroduction would be of great public benefit.

A fragrant smell is as much a factor in health as in beauty, and part of the curative effect of essences may be seen in the subtle change in odour which they bring about, for this is normally an indication of structural change. This idea is confirmed in practice. Take, for instance, the example of phenols and alcohols. Phenols possess the property of attaching themselves to the amino-acids which cause the destructive action of numerous microbial germs or their secretions, as well as tissual waste in wounds, burns and skin conditions. The resulting products (aminophenols) are well-known for their antiseptic action – in fact, this is one of the explanations of the bactericidal action of phenols. Alcohols behave in a similar fashion, producing amino-alcohols. Amino-menthol and other amino-alcohols have been linked with *certain* substances which are active with regard to the leprosy bacillus, parent of the tubercle bacillus – and this would explain the action of menthol on bronchial patients. The picture is similar for aldehydes, in particular citral.

We have already considered the healing power of aromatic essences in relation to burns and wounds, in that they encourage the reconstruction of damaged tissue. *Skin diseases* too will sometimes respond to treatment with essential oils. Lesions of this kind are always a sign of a poor organic condition and indicate abnormality in the composition of the layers of the skin and the presence of an element of decay. Besides halting the decay, essences may encourage a synthesis which leads to the reconstruction of the tissue. The various dermatoses (wet or dry), acne and blotches are curable by both local and *general* treatment with essences. Local application of essences also acts upon the subjacent organ (liver, intestine, circulatory system) whose deficiency has given rise to the cutaneous problem.

Apart from citral (either in ointment form or injected), and various pastes which may be neutral or acid, there are special combinations of flower essences (from both indigenous and exotic flowers) which may be used in the treatment of eczema and indeed a variety of skin conditions, particularly acne, certain types of psoriasis, "bricklayers' itch" and the butterfly mask of pregnancy. While such essences as mustard, cinnamon, cloves, turpentine, pine and cypress are strongly rubefacient, the majority have only a slight irritant action on the skin and deterpenated essences none at all.

Pediculosis (lousiness) and *scabies* are alleviated by medications based on essential oils. A drop of lavender, lemon, rosemary, orange flower, cloves, cinnamon, mustard or thyme will kill the scabies mite (*Sarcoptes scabiei*) in a few minutes; this was verified by microscopic examination by Delafond and Bourguignon in 1862. Many such formulae will be found elsewhere in this book.

The *pesticidal* properties of essences have also been known since antiquity. The essences of lavender, geranium and origanum, among others, will repel insects including moths and mosquitoes and are wonderfully effective in the treatment of insect bites, spider bites and wasp stings.

In fact most essences have *antitoxic* and *antivenomous* properties. In the case of these bites and stings, if one has no bottle of essence to hand, an excellent substitute treatment is to rub the affected parts with the flowers of lavender or rosemary, sage leaves, a cut leek or a piece of onion or garlic. The pain quickly disappears and the inflammation fades away within a few minutes (one should not of course forget to remove a wasp's sting in due course). These essences neutralise the insect venom; in fact, we have here a phenomenon of considerable importance, since the venom is neutralised by the significant diffusion of the essences.[3]

L. Binet reminds us that broom also neutralises venoms; sheep which have chewed broom are found to be resistant to adder bites. G. Billard has demonstrated that when a solution of spartein sulphate (the active principle of broom) is mixed with adder venom, the venom is rendered harmless.

Many essential oils have *anti-neuralgic* and *antirheumatic* properties when applied to a localised area in the form of emulsions, ointments, liniments or compresses. This knowledge has been used for centuries; in the past people used applications of plants they heated in the oven or poultices of garlic, onion, thyme and sage to treat painful rheumatic conditions and gout.

The antirheumatic properties, then, are released by external use and act on a particular area. But the large-scale diffusion of essences through the skin suggests that the treatment also works generally. In my earlier discussion of aromatic baths, I mentioned that recent research had

3   The diffusibility of essences is astonishing. As I mentioned in an earlier book, it is enough to shave a small area of a guinea-pig's head and rub it with a little essence of lavender for the kidneys of the animal to smell of lavender at a post-mortem only half an hour later. This applies whether the essences are introduced through the bone, intra-muscularly, intravenously, through the rectum or vagina, or by inhalation.

proved that essences pass through the layers of the skin to be rapidly circulated in the blood, and then eliminated via the lungs and kidneys in particular. The organs benefit from the disinfectant, antispasmodic or stimulant properties of the essences in the process. Juniper baths are recommended for people suffering from rheumatism or arthritis; baths of marjoram, thyme, rosemary or sage are fortifying, baths of lavender are soothing, as also are baths of lime flowers. The reader will find various applications of general and localised bathing under the studies of individual essences.

The skin's absorptiveness has always been exploited in the treatment of general conditions (e.g. with iodine paint or friction rubbing with liniments based on garlic, olive oil or camphor). The modern pharmacopoeia contains many ointments whose active principle (anti-coagulant or hormonal), is designed to have an effect on the whole body through rubbing into the skin.

Some years ago Professor C. Vallette[4] made a study of the ability of essences to penetrate the skin. Soluble in skin grease, they were found to pass quickly through the external layers and into the blood. High doses of essential oils applied to the skins of mice or rats caused immediate death, lower doses producing either depression or exaltation. He studied comparative rates of penetration by plucking the abdomen of a rabbit and applying 1/100cc of essence to a circular area 3cm in diameter, over which he then placed a watch glass, fixing it to the skin with glue. All that then remained was to record the moment when the last trace of liquid disappeared. This experiment produced the following results: essence of turpentine was absorbed in 20 minutes; thyme and eucalyptus in 20–40 minutes; bergamot, lemon and anise in 40–60 minutes; citronella, pine, lavender, cinnamon and geranium in 60–70 minutes, and the essences of mint, coriander and rue in approximately 100 minutes.

It will be apparent that, apart from the effects they themselves have, essences may act as a support or as carriers for a variety of other medicaments applied locally to obtain general effects (e.g. alkaloids and various glucosides). This explains why a solution of 1 centigram of morphine in eucalyptol applied externally to the abdomen of a rabbit will in three minutes cause a reduction in the respiration rate, which also becomes irregular. A solution of 4.5 milligrams of strychnine sulphate used in the same way will produce convulsions in 25 minutes and death two hours later. The mixture obtained with only 2cg of pilocarpine hydrochlorate produces defecation after 20 minutes. We can therefore say with certainty that aromatic essences applied to the skin affect the underlying organs.

If essences have this effect when applied to a local area of the skin, one wonders immediately how powerfully they must act when taken internally. In fact their properties are varying and almost infinite when taken in

4 C. Valette: *Pénétration transcutanée des essences* (C. R. Soc. Biologique, 1945).

this way. All are indicated in more than one set of circumstances, which makes it very difficult to classify them according to their therapeutic properties.

They are found to be antiseptics (with regard to lungs, intestine and urinary tract), anti-ferments, detoxifiers, remineralisers, stimulants and antispasmodics (not in fact incompatible, since essences are usually *balancing agents*), diuretics, antirheumatics, digestives, carminatives, febrifuges, cholagogues and vermifuges. The majority have hormonal properties which act on the cortex of the suprarenal (adrenal) glands, ovaries and thyroid. Some are aphrodisiacs, able, according to Roques, to "revitalise organs worn out with old age or jaded by dissolute living"; others have been shown to be vaso-dilators or vaso-constrictors and to act against diabetes.

As a result of a great deal of research, we are now able to explain, for instance, the action of essences on the intestinal motor function, their relations with the various endocrine glands, the manner in which they are eliminated and their vascular, analgesic and cell-protecting properties.

Among the *antiseptics* we may mention lemon, thyme, lavender, turpentine, pine, eucalpytus, cloves, etc – in fact the list is almost endless. In the treatment of tuberculosis, the use of essential oils brings about a lowering of temperature, a reduction in coughing, the regaining of appetite, weight and strength, a normalisation of blood-counts (particularly sedimentation rate) and the disappearance of the tubercle bacillus and scar cavities.

Rosemary aids the production and evacuation of *bile*; the essences of lavender, mint, sage and thyme are also choleretic.[5]

Garlic, hyssop, juniper, lemon, nutmeg and onion are prophylactic with regard to the formation of biliary or urinary calculi.

Lavender, marjoram, lemongrass, cypress and anise have *antispasmodic* properties. A few drops of essence of tarragon on the tongue will instantly stop hiccoughs; some drops of essence of cypress on the pillow will rapidly control a spasmodic cough; lavender calms an overexcited nervous system.

Most essences are *stimulants*. The essences of pine (needles), borneol, geranium, basil, sage, savory and rosemary dynamise the cortex of the suprarenal (adrenal) gland; anise excites the anterior pituitary body, as does mint; onion, garlic and lemon are tonics. Onion, cinnamon, borneol, savory and ylang-ylang can help those whose sexual faculties are waning, whereas camphor has anaphrodisiac properties. Camomile, garlic, onion and cinnamon are sudorifics.

I have already mentioned the healing properties of lavender, sage, rosemary and thyme, as applied externally: they are also widely used in the treatment of colitis, which is so prevalent today. As to their detoxify-

---

5   R. Cazal: *Contribution à l'étude de l'activité pharmacodynamique de quelques essences de labiées* (Thetis-Toulouse, 1944).

ing properties, these can be put to daily use fighting the numerous forms of poisoning (alimentary and medicinal) to which man is currently subject.

Those aromatic essences I discussed in relation to their effect on burns and infected and gangrenous wounds possess the same antitoxic power when administered internally.

Garlic, onion, anise, lemon, juniper and thyme act against *fermentations* – and one should not forget the major role played by intestinal infection in the flare-up of the majority of diseases, cancer included. The daily ingestion of aromatics guarantees proper balance and functioning of the intestines. Patients who treat themselves with plants and essences and regularly use aromatics in their food all acknowledge that their stools become deodorised: putrefaction, so dangerous in the long run, is unknown. A 24-hour fast followed by the ingestion for a further 24 hours to 48 hours of essential oils leads to such a bodily and intestinal disinfection that stools take on an aromatic odour.

Numerous essences are *vermifuge*. Without listing them all, I will mention garlic, camomile, lemon, thyme, onion, wormseed, bergamot, caraway, cinnamon and geraniol.

Sage, cypress and lemongrass have *hormonal* porperties, the essence of cypress being a homologue of the ovarian hormone. These have a balancing effect on the endocrine glands and operate by dynamising and giving them new impetus rather than taking over the functions of deficient glands. This means that aromatic essences play a role of prime importance in the sphere of physiological excitation therapy. The properties of the onion with regard to normalising glandular imbalance and obesity are well known.

Among those essences which normalise and promote the *menstrual cycle* (emmenagogics) mention should be made of rue, valerian, artemisia, basil, cinnamon, cumin, lavender, melissa, mint, savin, clary and thyme.

The following lower *arterial pressure*: lavender, aspic (by peripheral action in lowering superficial blood pressure) and marjoram (by a central mechanism). The essences of hyssop, rosemary, sage and thyme on the other hand raise arterial pressure by liberating adrenalin as a result of direct action on the area of the cortex of the adrenal gland.

Anise, caraway, fennel and lemongrass increase the size of the breasts and promote *lactation*, whereas parsley, mint and sage reduce the milk-supply.

The *antidiabetic* properties of eucalyptus, onion and geranium could well be put to profitable use since, as American research has shown[6] the

---

6 *United States – Frequency of Diabetes.* A group of American doctors undertook a study of the incidence of diabetes among the population of Oxford, Massachusetts. Their results, which accord with those of British doctors, indicated that diabetes is commoner and more dangerous than had been suspected, showing an incidence of 1.7% as opposed to the generally admitted percentage of between 0.1 and 0.4%.

incidence of diabetes is rising; in fact their use ought to become quite automatic.

Other plants with similar properties include leaves of walnut, myrtle, mulberry and olive, agrimony, burdock, knotgrass, goatsrue and figwort.

To close this list – which could truly go on for ever – let me draw attention to the *diuretic* properties of fennel root, which Dioscorides recommended to "those who can only piss a drop at a time", and various essences including, in particular, juniper and onion. There is a story about a government minister who wanted personal proof that the reported diuretic powers of the onion were not somewhat exaggerated; he made himself an alcoholic maceration of onion juice which he then swallowed. Unfortunately it happened to be a period of important parliamentary activity; he had no choice but to keep interrupting his working sessions to answer the calls of nature. Antirheumatic properties are linked with the diuretic properties of these essences (again, these may be found in other plants). Their ability to eliminate uric acid could be put to good use by many patients.

There have been many people who, faced with the evidence of the different properties I have listed, have presented a variety of theories in their attempts to discover exactly *how* the aromatic essences work; numerous explanations have been put forward. I will describe a few of these here, starting with Filatob's theory of "biogen stimulation" which is based on the idea that a living tissue (human, animal or vegetable) separated from its organism and kept in conditions of *suffering* (cold, desiccation, *distillation*) will produce certain substances of resistance in its struggle to survive, viz the bio-or phyto-stimulines. Introduced into a deficient organism, these substances will reactivate the failing vital processes and, strengthening the cellular metabolism, improve the various physiological functions, at the same time fighting infection and stimulating the regeneration of tissue.

From a different viewpoint, aromatic essences have been compared to vegetable *hormones*; we have already seen that the essence of cypress seems to be the homologue of the ovarian hormone and that essence of pine needles, and other essences, will stimulate the cortex of the adrenal gland.

Perner and Zenife demonstrated in a detailed study the effects of a number of different plants on the menstrual cycle.[7]

Further studies offer strong evidence to support the supposition that essences are able to act upon and modify the patient's *electro-magnetic field*. There are also authors who hold that plant extracts have a vibratory effect on the vagosympathetic system – this theory is frequently invoked with regard to biological phenomena and to the maintenance or re-establishment of health. The works of Laville and de Lakhowsky throw particular light on this hypothesis.

7 Perner – Zenife: *Les phyto-hormones et l'activité oestrogène de certains végétaux* (Revue Pharmaceutique Tchécoslovaque, 1959).

Lastly, reference to my own work[8] will afford at least a partial explanation of the action of essences in terms of their pH value, their rH_2 and their resistance.

Since it is no part of this present book to elaborate complex physico-chemical notions, I shall give a simplified account.

The pH represents, by a figure, the acidity or alkalinity of a solution. It varies between 0 and 14.14; the weaker the pH value, the more acid the solution. Pure water is 7.07. Vitamins have an acid reaction less than 6 or 5 – fruit and fruit juices of low pH value are sources of vitamin. Wine ferments in an acid medium, as does milk when it turns into yogurt, a powerful intestinal disinfectant. On the other hand, rotten eggs and bad meat produce an alkaline reaction. This is why we keep gherkins in vinegar, which is acid, rather than in, say, Vichy water, which is an alkaline.

The rH_2 factor defines the charge in electrons of a given pH value (for the same pH value there will be an infinite number of rH_2 values) and the power of oxido-reduction, i.e. the balance between the phenomena of oxidation and reduction, which will vary according to circumstance. The rH_2 table runs from 0 to 42. The rH_2 values are extremely slight: a value of 28 (a balance between the pressures of oxygen or hydrogen) represents a theoretical pressure of oxygen or hydrogen of one ten-thousand-millionth of a ten-thousand-millionth of a ten-thousand-millionth of an atmosphere.

Thirdly, resistance is the property of a solution to oppose transmission of heat or electricity. The purer a solution, the less conductive it is to the transmission of electricity. The resistance of blood is on average 190 ohms/cm/cm^2 for a man, 220/230 for a woman.

Generally speaking, natural essences have an acid pH value and, which is important, high resistance. For instance, the resistance of essence of cloves is measured at 4,000 (20 times that of human blood), thyme at 3,300, lavender at 2,800 and mint at 3,000. A mixture of essences which, as we have seen, has strong bactericidal properties through nebulisation in the atmosphere, has a resistance of 17,000 – thus the resistance of the mixture is much greater than that of its component essences. Its pH is very acid, at 4.6. Alkalinity favours the rapid multiplication of microbes whereas acidity opposes it, hence the bactericidal properties of the essences. The high resistance of essences also discourages the diffusion of infections and toxins.

The rH_2 (potential of oxido-reduction) has a value which varies according to the essence and activates the oxidation or reduces it accordingly. The antimicrobial properties of peppermint, which is also a powerful oxidising agent, may thus be explained. Conversely, essence of cloves is a reductive agent, and therefore displays antiviral and anti-

---

8   e.g. Dr Jean Valnet and Claude Reddet: *Contribution à l'application pratique d'une nouvelle conception du terrain biologique* (A.M.I.F. Avril–Mai 1961).

carcinogenic properties.[9] Microbial conditions in general correspond to a state of alkalinity with fairly low rH_2 and a correspondingly low resistance. But, as always, practice is not quite as simple as theory. Charles Nicolle said, "One should not try to constrain any biological method in a formula. Sooner or later the facts will break out."

Before we turn to the particular uses of specific essences, let us take a final look at the different methods, both external and internal, by which they may be administered.

Externally, they may be used pure or in the form of a soapy or aqueous emulsion, in an alcoholic solution, as a liniment, or indeed in overall or localised bathing. They are also frequently used as enemas, vaginal douches, inhalations or aerosols. Finally, they may be administerd in the form of injections. I undertook with my colleagues a series of wide-ranging tests on various mixtures of whole natural aromatic essences in emulsion form for use in ordinary bathing and washing. The mixture for adults contained the essences of cypress, lavender, rosemary, sage and thyme; the mixture for children included the essences of lavender, rosemary, thyme, savory and origanum, and for old people the mixture contained lavender, thyme, juniper, geranium and wild thyme. The effects – tonic or calming, decongestive or balancing – were experienced after only a few baths or washes. Knowledge of the constituents of these essences clarifies why cases of obesity, cellulitis, arthrosis, circulatory problems, muscular weakness, insomnia and nervousness benefit from aromatic baths taken as a form of general treatment.

The diffusiblity of the essences means, as we saw earlier, that they will act as vectors, i.e. agents of penetration. They have for a long time been produced in the form of creams, balms and lotions so that their active principles might be diffused easily throughout the body. Thus the action of seaweed baths is necessarily reinforced and completed by the addition of certain essences, which, as vegetable hormones, are complementary in any case. Practice has confirmed this theory, and various mixtures of aromatic herbs are now used in association with seaweed to dynamise the familiar effects of seaweed baths.[10]

Internally, the essential oils are prescribed in the form of either capsules or drops or, most often, in honey water. They are given alone or in association with other oils. Depending on the case, dosage will vary between 5 and 20 drops of pure essence administered several times a day before or during meals, or between 20 and 30 drops taken four times a day in honey diluted in half a glass of warm water (see Chapter 8).

9   According to L. Cl. Vincent, cancerous forms are accompanied by an alkaline pH value, by a high rH_2 value (above 25–26) and by lowered resistance (below 170 and down to 110 or 100, the point of no return). The essence of cloves has an acid pH value (6.7), a low rH_2 value (16.5) and a very high resistance (4,000), and has been found to have electronic constituents which are opposed to cancer and to virus diseases.

10   These bath-essences – *Alg-Essences* – are produced by Lab Marins – BP 23 – 45300 Pithivers, France.

Since their effects are powerful, it is usually necessary to administer them in very diluted solutions. The polarimetric charge of a solution of essential oil is in inverse proportion to its richness in essences, i.e. in certain cases one obtains more effective results when the product is more dilute (we are not talking here of homoeopathy).

Care should be taken when essences are used which contain ketones, for in certain doses they may be epilepsy-inducing in patients so predisposed. The essences of rosemary, fennel,[11] hyssop, wormwood and sage fall into this category, whereas anise, burdock, melissa, mint and origanum are, according to Cadéac and Meunier, liable to be stupefacient under certain conditions (chiefly if over-used).

There are "scientists" who will deny to the bitter end the facts before their eyes; it is they who have denied aromatherapy the right to be treated as a branch of science. But there have always been other scientists who have revolted against this attitude, which, after all, is plainly in opposition to the true scientific spirit.

11   In experiments the essences of fennel and rosemary have been found to render animals nervous, while essences of wormwood, hyssop and sage render them aggressive.

PART TWO

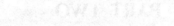

Chapter 1

A Essences classified by their principal properties

ANALGESIC (pain-relieving): cajuput, camomile, cinnamon, clove, coriander, garlic, geranium, ginger, lavender, marjoram, niaouli, nutmeg, onion, origanum, peppermint, rosemary, sage, terebinth

ANTIANAEMIC: camomile, lemon, thyme (in infants)

ANTIARTHRITIC: garlic, lemon

ANTICANCER: clove, cypress, hyssop, garlic, geranium, (onion), sage, (tarragon), thuja

ANTIDIABETIC: eucalyptus, geranium, juniper, onion

ANTIDIARRHOEIC: camomile, cinnamon, clove, garlic, geranium, ginger, lavender, lemon, nutmeg, onion, orange blossom, peppermint, rosemary, sage, sandalwood, savory

ANTIDYSENTERY: cajuput, garlic, lemon, niaouli, thyme

ANTI-EPIDEMIC: see ANTI-INFECTION

ANTI-GALLSTONES: lemon, mace (nutmeg), onion, pine, rosemary, terebinth

ANTIGOUT: basil, cajuput, camomile, fennel, garlic, juniper, lemon, pine, rosemary, terebinth, thyme

ANTI-INFECTION: Borneo camphor, clove, eucalyptus, garlic, juniper, lavender, lemon, niaouli, pine, thyme

ANTI-INFLUENZAL: Borneo camphor, camomile, cinnamon, cypress, eucalyptus, hyssop, garlic, lavender, lemon, niaouli, peppermint, pine, rosemary, sage, thyme

ANTI-GALACTAGOGUE: peppermint, sage

ANTIMALARIAL: eucalyptus, lemon

ANTIMIGRAINE: lavender (and see Therapeutic Index)

ANTINEURALGIC, see ANALGESIC

ANTIOBESITY: lemon, onion

ANTIDONTALGIC (toothache): cajuput, cinnamon, clove, juniper (cade oil), nutmeg, onion, peppermint, sage

ANTIOPHTHALMIA: camomile

ANTIPHOLOGISTIC: camomile

ANTIPRURIGINOUS: camomile, lemon, menthol (peppermint)

ANTIRACHITIC (rickets): onion, pine, sage

ANTIRHEUMATIC: cajuput, camomile, cypress, eucalyptus, garlic, hyssop, juniper, lavender, lemon, niaouli, onion, origanum, pine, rosemary, sage, tarragon, terebinth, thuja, thyme

ANTISCLEROTIC: garlic, lemon, onion

ANTISCORBUTIC: ginger, lemon, onion

ANTISEPTIC, GENERAL: basil, bergamot, Borneo camphor, cajuput, camomile, cinnamon, clove, eucalyptus, garlic, geranium, ginger, hyssop, juniper, lavender, lemon, lemongrass, niaouli, nutmeg, onion, origanum, peppermint, pine, rosemary, sage, savory, terebinth, thyme, ylang-ylang

> HEPATIC: pine
>
> INTESTINAL: basil, bergamot, cajuput, cinnamon, garlic, geranium, ginger, juniper, lavender, lemon, lemongrass, niaouli, nutmeg, onion, peppermint, rosemary, sage, savory, thyme, ylang-ylang
>
> PULMONARY: cajuput, clove, eucalyptus, garlic, hyssop, juniper, lavender, lemon, niaouli, onion, origanum, peppermint, pine, rosemary, sage, sandalwood, terebinth, thyme
>
> URINARY: cajuput, eucalyptus, juniper, lavender, lemon, niaouli, onion, pine, sage, sandalwood, terebinth, thyme

ANTISPASMODIC: aniseed, basil, bergamot, cajuput, camomile, caraway, cinnamon, clove, cypress, fennel, garlic, hyssop, lavender, lavender-cotton, lemon, marjoram, nutmeg, onion, origanum, peppermint, rosemary, sage, savory, terebinth, thyme

ANTISUDORAL: sage

ANTITHROMBOSIS: onion

ANTITOXIC: lemon

ANTITUSSIVE: hyssop, lavender, rosemary

ANTIVENOMOUS: lavender, lemon

ANTI-URINARY STONES: fennel, garlic, geranium, hyssop, juniper, lemon, terebinth

APERITIF (Appetite stimulant): camomile, caraway, fennel, garlic, ginger, origanum, sage, tarragon, thyme

APHRODISIAC: aniseed (?), cinnamon, clove, ginger, juniper, lemongrass, onion, peppermint, pine, rosemary, sandalwood, savory, thyme, ylang-ylang

ASTRINGENT: cinammon, cypress, geranium, lemon, sage, sandalwood

BACTERICIDES: camomile, garlic, lavender, lemon (and see Individual Studies)

BACTERIOSTATIC: camomile, garlic

BALSAMIC: eucalyptus, niaouli, pine, terebinth, thyme

BLOOD-THINNING: garlic, lemon

CALMATIVE: aniseed, basil, bergamot, cajuput, camomile, cinnamon, cypress, garlic, lavender, marjoram, sage

CARMINATIVE: aniseed, caraway, cinnamon, clove, coriander, fennel, garlic, ginger, lemon, marjoram, nutmeg, origanum, peppermint, rosemary, savory, thyme

CAUSTIC: clove

CHOLAGOGUES: camomile, lavender, rosemary

CICATRISING: (aiding formation of scar-tissue, healing): cajuput, camomile, clove, eucalyptus, garlic, geranium, hyssop, juniper, lavender, lavandin, lemon, niaouli, onion, rosemary, sage, savory, terebinth, thyme

COUNTER-IRRITANT, see REVULSIVE

DEODORANT: cypress

DEPURATIVE: lemon, juniper, sage

DIURETIC: aniseed, caraway, cypress, fennel, garlic, hyssop, juniper, lavender, lemon, onion, rosemary, sage, terebinth, thuja, thyme

EMMENAGOGUES: basil, camomile, caraway, cinnamon, fennel, hyssop, juniper, lavender, lavender-cotton, nutmeg, origanum, peppermint, rosemary, sage, thyme

EXPECTORANTS: eucalyptus, fennel, hyssop, lavender, marjoram, onion, origanum, peppermint, pine, savory, terebinth, thuja, thyme

FEBRIFUGES: camomile, eucalyptus, garlic, ginger, lemon

GALACTAGOGUES: aniseed, caraway (?), fennel, lemongrass

HAEMOSTATIC: cinnamon, cypress, geranium, juniper, lemon, terebinth

HEALING, see CICATRISING

HYPERTENSIVE: hyssop, rosemary, sage, thyme

HYPNOTIC: basil, camomile, lavender, marjoram, onion (mild), orange blossom (mild), thyme (mild)

HYPOTENSIVE: garlic, lavender, lemon, marjoram, ylang-ylang

PARASITICIDES: caraway, cinnamon, clove, eucalyptus, garlic, geranium, juniper, lavender, lemon, lemongrass, origanum, peppermint, rosemary, terebinth, thyme

RESOLVENT: fennel, garlic, hyssop, onion, rosemary, savory

RESTORATIVE, GENERAL AND OF THE NERVES: basil, cypress, lavender, marjoram, rosemary,

    GLANDULAR: garlic, onion

REVULSIVE: terebinth, thyme

RUBEFACIENT: pine

SEDATIVE: camomile, lavender, lemon, marjoram, thyme

STIMULANTS, GENERAL: aniseed, Borneo camphor, camomile, clove, coriander, eucalyptus, fennel, garlic, geranium, ginger, juniper, lavender, lavender-cotton, nutmeg, onion, peppermint, rosemary, sage, tarragon, thyme

    OF ADRENAL CORTEX: basil, Borneo camphor, geranium, pine, rosemary, sage, savory

    APPETITE, SEE *APERITIF*

    BULBAR: hyssop

CARDIAC (CARDIOTONIC): aniseed, Borneo camphor, caraway, cinnamon, garlic, lavender, lemon, rosemary

CEREBRAL (MENTAL AND MEMORY): basil, clove, nutmeg, onion, rosemary, savory, thyme

CIRCULATORY: caraway, cinnamon, garlic, nutmeg, thyme

DIGESTIVE: aniseed, camomile, caraway, cinnamon, fennel, garlic, hyssop, juniper, lemongrass, marjoram, nutmeg, onion, savory, tarragon (and see under STOMACHIC)

GASTRIC: bergamot (and see under STOMACHIC)

HEPATIC: lemon, onion

OF NERVOUS SYSTEM: basil, fennel, juniper, lemon, onion, peppermint, rosemary, sage, thyme

PANCREATIC: lemon

RENAL: onion

RESPIRATORY: aniseed, cinnamon, garlic

OF PRODUCTION OF WHITE CORPUSCLES: camomile, lemon, thyme

STOMACHIC: aniseed, basil, caraway, cinnamon, clove, coriander, garlic, ginger, hyssop, juniper, marjoram, nutmeg, onion, origanum, peppermint, rosemary, sage, savory, tarragon, thyme

SUDORIFIC: camomile, hyssop, juniper, lavender, rosemary, thuja, thyme

TONICS, GENERAL: Borneo camphor, garlic, lavender, peppermint, sage (see otherwise under STIMULANTS)

FOR SYMPATHETIC NERVOUS SYSTEM: lemon

UTERINE: clove

VENOUS: cypress, lemon

VASOCONSTRICTOR: cypress

VASODILATORS: garlic, marjoram

VERMIFUGES: bergamot, cajuput, camomile, caraway, cinnamon, clove, eucalyptus, fennel, garlic, hyssop, lavender, lavender-cotton, lemon, niaouli, onion, peppermint, savory, tarragon, terebinth, thuja, thyme .

VULNERARY: camomile, garlic, marjoram (and see under CICATRISING)

B   Principal Indications
(The most important indications are printed in italics)

Aniseed:
aerophagy, flatulence
nervous dyspepsia, nervous vomiting
infantile colic
migraine with nausea and vertigo
palpitations, false angina pectoris
asthma, bronchial spasm, cough, difficulty in breathing
painful menstrual periods
lacteal insufficiency

Basil:
nervous debility (mental fatigue)
anxiety, nervous insomnia
gastric and intestinal spasm, painful digestion
whooping cough, spasmodic cough
migraine, some types of vertigo
gout
scanty menstrual periods
paralysis, epilepsy (?)
external use: loss of sense of smell due to chronic catarrh

Bergamot:
general antiseptic and antispasmodic
loss of appetite, dyspepsia
intestinal colic
intestinal parasites

Borneo Camphor (borneol):
prophylaxis and treatment of *infectious diseases*, influenza
depressive states and debility (stimulates cortex of adrenal gland)
convalescence

Cajuput:
enteritis, dysentery
cystitis, urethritis
chronic pulmonary diseases (bronchitis, tuberculosis)
laryngitis, pharyngitis
gastric spasm
asthma
nervous vomiting
hysteria, epilepsy (?)
painful menstrual periods
rheumatism, gout
intestinal parasites

external uses: chronic laryngitis, rheumatic neuralgia, sores, skin diseases (acne, psoriasis), earache, toothache

Camomile:
loss of appetite
migraine
neuralgia (chiefly *facial)*
painful teething in infants
menopausal problems
vertigo, insomnia
painful digestion, stomach and intestinal cramps in children, infantile diarrhoea, enteritis
stomach ulcers, intestinal ulcers
anaemia
nervous depression, convulsions
scanty or *painful menstrual periods* linked with a nervous condition, amenorrhoea
influenzal headaches and pains in the lumbar region (backache)
intestinal parasites (roundworm, threadworm)
intermittent fevers, especially in patients suffering from nervous conditions

external uses: conjunctivitis, inflammation of the eyelids, inflamed skin conditions, eczema, herpes, boils, pruritis, sores, burns, rheumatic pains, gout

Caraway:
nervous dyspepsia, gastric spasm, indigestion
loss of appetite
flatulence, *aerophagy*
cardio-vascular erethism
intestinal parasites
difficult menstrual periods
lacteal insufficiency

external use: mange (in dogs)

Cinammon:
debility (especially influenzal)
fainting
sluggish digestion, gastric pain, flatulence
digestive spasm, spasmodic colitis
diarrhoea, putrefactive fermentations
uterine haemorrhage, haemoptysis (spitting blood)
scanty menstrual periods, leucorrhoea
impotence, frigidity
intestinal parasites

external uses: scabies, lice, wasp stings, contusions (aromatic tincture of arnica), toothache

Clove:
general physical and mental debility, amnesia
impotence (?)
difficult digestion, dyspepsia, flatulence, diarrhoea
pulmonary diseases (tuberculosis)
prevention of infectious diseases
intestinal parasites
preparation for childbirth
malignant conditions (?)

external uses: toothache, sores, ulcers, scabies, lupus, insect repellent, care of teeth

Coriander:
aerophagy, flatulence, painful digestion
loss of appetite
digestive spasm

external use: rheumatic neuralgia

Cypress:
haemorrhoids, varicose veins
ovarian disorders (painful menstrual periods, uterine haemorrhage)
menopausal problems
whooping cough, spasmodic cough, aphonia (loss of voice)
spasms
influenza
enuresis
rheumatism
irritability (general restorative, especially of the nervous system)
malignant conditions (?)

external uses: haemorrhoids, offensive sweating of the feet

Eucalyptus:
diseases of the respiratory tract: acute and chronic bronchitis, cough, influenza, pulmonary tuberculosis, gangrene, asthma, pneumonia

diseases of the urinary tract: various infections, *colibacillosis*, cystitis
diabetes
*various feverish complaints and infections: measles, scarlet fever (pro-
    phylactic); cholera, malaria, typhus*
rheumatism, neuralgia
intestinal parasites (roundworm, threadworm)
migraine
general debility

external uses: sores, burns (cicatrising), lice, mosquito repellent, domes-
    tic disinfectant

Fennel
flatulence, sluggish digestion, gastralgia (stomach pains)
aerophagy, loss of appetite, *nervous vomiting*
oliguria, urinary stones, gout
scanty menstrual periods
pulmonary diseases, influenza (prophylactic)
lacteal insufficiency
intestinal parasites

external uses: congestion of the breasts, bruises, tumours, deafness

Garlic
*prophylaxis and treatment of infectious diseases (epidemics of influenza,
    typhoid, diphtheria)*
asthma, emphysema (modifies bronchial secretions)
diseases of the respiratory tract: bronchitis, *tuberculosis*, pulmonary
    gangrene, *whooping cough*, influenza, colds
arterial hypertension
arteriosclerosis, senescence (ageing)
rheumatism, gout, arthritis
urinary stones
gonorrhoea
dysentery, diarrhoea, intestinal infections
intestinal parasites (roundworm, threadworm, tapeworm)
malignant conditions, (preventive, by anti-putrid intestinal action ?)

external uses: corns, warts, verrucas, callouses, wounds, ulcers, scabies,
    tinea, deafness, earache, rheumatic neuralgia, insect bites, cold abscesses

Geranium:
debility (resulting from deficiency of cortex of adrenal gland)
gastro-enteritis, diarrhoea
uterine and pulmonary haemorrhage (decoction of leaves)
sterility

jaundice
diabetes (decoction of leaves)
urinary stones
gastric ulcer
cancer of the uterus (?)

external uses: sores, burns, congestion of breasts, inflammation of mouth and tongue, sore throat, tonsillitis, facial neuralgia, ophthalmia, impotence (?), lumbar and gastric pains, scurf, dry eczema, lice

Ginger:
loss of apetite
painful digestion, flatulence
diarrhoea
scurvy

external use: rheumatic pains

Hyssop:
asthma, hay fever, pulmonary emphysema, difficulty in breathing
chronic bronchitis, cough, influenza
loss of appetite, painful digestion
gastralgia, colic
rheumatism
leucorrhoea, scanty menstrual periods
urinary stones
intestinal parasites
malignant conditions (?)

external uses: dermatosis, eczema, sores, bruises

Juniper:
general debility; organic lassitude (sluggish digestion)
prophylactic of contagious diseases
diseases of the urinary tract: albuminuria, oliguria, gonorrhoea, cystitis
gout
rheumatism, arthritis
urinary stones
diabetes
dropsy, cirrhosis
arteriosclerosis
leucorrhoea, painful and difficult menstrual periods
flatulence

external uses: after-effects of paralysis, sores, ulcers, weeping eczema, acne, toothache (Cade oil), domestic disinfectant, canine mange

Lavender:
irritability, spasm, insomnia

87

diseases of the respiratory tract: asthma, bronchitis (acute), *spasmodic cough (whooping cough), influenza*, etc
eruptive fevers, infectious diseases
scrofulosis (ganglions)
general physical and mental debility, anxiety, melancholy
infantile debility
migraine, vertigo, hysteria, epilepsy, *after-effects of paralysis*
enteritis (diarrhoea), dyspepsia, sluggish digestion, gastric atony
cystitis, *gonorrhoea*
oliguria
leucorrhoea, scanty menstrual periods
intestinal parasites

external uses: the treatment of wounds of all descriptions, burns, acne, eczema, lice, scabies, *insect bites*, animal and snake bites; used also in inhalations and as a domestic disinfectant

Lavender-cotton
intestinal parasites (roundworm, threadworm)
spasm
scanty menstrual periods

Lemon:
various infections, infectious diseases, epidemics (prophylaxis and treatment)
debility, loss of appetite
rheumatism, arthritis, gout
gastric hyperacidity, stomach ulcers
arteriosclerosis, hypertension
varicose veins, phlebitis, capillary fragility
plethora, hyperviscosity of the blood
ascites (dropsy of the abdomen)
urinary stones, gallstones
demineralisation, growing pains, convalescence, pulmonary tuberculosis, tuberculosis of the spine (Pott's disease)
anaemia
scurvy
jaundice, *hepatic congestion, hepatic deficiency*
painful digestion, vomiting
haemorrhage (nasal, gastric, intestinal, renal)
diarrhoea
malaria, feverish conditions
intestinal parasites
equally: asthma, bronchitis, influenza, haemophilia, gonorrhoea, syphilis, senescence, headache

external uses: inflammations of mouth and tongue, thrush, buccal syphilides, infected and putrid wounds, verrucas, warts, herpes, tinea, scabies, eruptions of various kinds, boils, insect bites

Lemongrass:
difficult digestion
enteritis, *colitis*
upsetting of sympathetic nervous system and resulting disorders (spasm, palpitations, vertigo, etc)
insufficiency of milk
external use: lice

Marjoram:
(properties similar to those of peppermint and thyme)
general debility
digestive spasm (aerophagy), flatulence
respiratory spasm
nervous debility, mental instability
migraine
anxiety, insomnia, tics
external uses: rheumatic neuralgia, head colds

Niaouli:
chronic and fetid bronchitis, pulmonary tuberculosis
whooping cough
rhinitis, sinusitis, otitis
tuberculosis of the bones
inestinal infections (enteritis, dysentery)
urinary infections (cystitis)
puerperal infections (after childbirth)

external uses: sores, *atonic wounds*, burns, fistulas, pulmonary diseases, laryngitis, whooping cough, coryza (cold in the head)

Nutmeg:
chronic diarrhoea
difficult digestion
halitosis, flatulence
debility
gallstones
external uses: rheumatic pains, toothache

Onion:
general debiltiy, physical and mental fatigue
growing pains

retention of liquid in system (oedema, pleurisy, ascites, dropsy, peri-carditis)
oliguria
rheumatism, arthritis
excess urea in blood
obesity
gallstones
diabetes
difficult and sluggish digestion
diarrhoea, *intestinal fermentation*
genito-urinary infections
respiratory diseases (colds, bronchitis, asthma, laryngitis)
glandular imbalance
arteriosclerosis, senescence (retards)
prostatitis, impotence
lymphatism, rickets
scurvy
intestinal parasites

external uses: abscess, boils, insect bites and wasp stings, chilblains, chaps, warts, deafness, haemorrhoids

Orange Blossom:
cardiac spasm, palpitations
chronic diarrhoea
insomnia

Origanum:
loss of appetite
sluggish digestion, gastric atony
aerophagy (digestive spasm), *flatulence*
chronic bronchitis, irritating cough
pulmonary tuberculosis
asthma
acute or chronic rheumatism, muscular rheumatism
amenorrhoea (absence of menstruation)

external uses: rheumatic pains, lice

Peppermint:
general debility
indigestion, gastric atony, aerophagy
stomach-ache, acidity of the stomach
flatulence, diarrhoea, cholera, gastro-intestinal poisoning
gastric spasm and colic
liver complaints
nervous vomiting
palpitations, vertigo

migraine, tremors, paralysis
difficult and *painful periods*
asthma, chronic bronchitis
impotence (mild action)
intestinal parasites

external uses: headache, migraine, toothache, scabies, mosquito repellent; used also in inhalations

Pine:
all diseases of respiratory tract (asthma, bronchitis, tuberculosis, tracheitis, etc)
urinary diseases (pyelitis, cystitis, prostatitis)
infections in general
gallstones
impotence
rickets
stomach-ache, intestinal pains

external uses: pulmonary complaints; generally in baths (rheumatism, gout, etc)

Rosemary:
general debility, physical and mental fatigue, amnesia
chlorosis, lymphatism
asthma, chronic bronchitis, whooping cough
intestinal infections, colitis, diarrhoea
flatulence, *difficult digestion*, stomach-ache
rheumatism, gout
hepatic disorders, jaundice, gallstones, cirrhosis, *cholecystitis*
excess of cholesterol in the blood
painful periods, leucorrhoea
migraine
disorders of the nervous system: *epilepsy, after-effects of paralysis*, weakness of limbs
cardiac complaints of nervous origin
vertigo, fainting, hysteria

external uses: sores, burns, lice, scabies; tonic and aphrodisiac baths; rheumatism

Sage:
(a general tonic to the system)
debility, (convalescence, etc), *nervous debility*
dyspepsia, sluggish digestion, loss of appetite
diarrhoea
nervous complaints: trembling, vertigo, paralysis
chronic bronchitis, asthma

nocturnal sweating in tubercular patients and convalescents
profuse sweating of hands and armpits
oliguria
lymphatism
hypotension
painful and *scanty periods*, *menopause*
preparation for childbirth
sterility
intermittent fevers
lactation (to dry up)

external uses: leucorrhoea, *thrush*, *stomatitis*, throat infections, tooth-ache, *atonic wounds*, eczema, insect bites and stings (wasps, etc), tonic baths, domestic disinfectant

Sandalwood:
specific for urinary infections: *gonorrhoea*, cystitis, colibacillosis
chronic bronchitis
persistent diarrhoea
impotence (?)

Savory:
painful digestion
mental fatigue
impotence
gastric pains of nervous origin
flatulence, intestinal fermentations
intestinal spasm
diarrhoea of all kinds
intestinal parasites
asthma, bronchitis
eye strain

external uses: sores, deafness
(one of the essences with the most active antibacterial and anti-fungal properties, See the section devoted specifically to it).

Tarragon:
upsets of the sympathetic nervous system (aerophagy, *hiccough*)
loss of appetite, sluggish digestion
stomach-ache, nervous dyspepsia
flatulence, putrefactive fermentations
rheumatic neuralgia
painful and difficult periods
intestinal parasites

Terebinth:
chronic and fetid *bronchitis*, pulmonary tuberculosis

92

urinary infections, cystitis, urethritis
leucorrhoea
haemorrhage (intestinal, pulmonary, uterine, nasal)
gallstones
spasms (colitis, whooping cough)
rheumatism, *gout*, neuralgia, sciatica
migraine
intestinal parasites (especially tapeworm)
chronic constipation
epilepsy
antidote to phosphorous poisoning

external uses: pulmonary diseases, rheumatic neuralgia (gout, sciatica), lice, scabies

Thuja:
cystitis, enlarged prostate, pelvic congestion
rheumatism

external uses: verrucas, warts, condylomas, adenoids (as a gargle)

Thyme:
general physical and mental debility, nervous debility, anaemia (in children)
chlorosis
asthma
spasmodic *cough* (whooping cough, etc)
pulmonary diseases (modifies secretions, antiseptic and antispasmodic)
sluggish digestion
intestinal infections (fermentations), *urinary infections*
diseases resulting from chill (*influenza*, colds, stiffness, shivering, sore throat, etc): *one of the best remedies*
infectious diseases
intestinal parasites (hookworm, roundworm, threadworm, tapeworm)
aids the circulation; indicated for unnatural *suppression* of periods
leucorrhoea
also aids *sleep*

external uses: dermatoses, boils, wounds, lice, scabies, vaginal douches, sprays (generally in association with other essences), care of teeth and gums, rheumatism

Ylang-ylang:
hypertension (high blood pressure)
tachycardia (acceleration of heartbeat)
intestinal infections
purulent secretions
impotence, frigidity

2. Studies of Individual Essences

(To simplify calculations of quantities, 1 gram of aromatic essence is roughly equal to 20 drops).

Aniseed

Pimpinella anisum

Umbelliferae

Parts used: seeds, essence.

Principal known constituents: an essence (anethol, methyl chavicol, terpenes), starch, sugar, choline, malic acid, resins.

Properties:
- *antispasmodic,* calmative
- *stomachic*
- *carminative*
- *general stimulant* (cardiac, respiratory, digestive); it acts at the same time as a sedative on these organs
- galactagogue
- diuretic
- aphrodisiac (?)
- *in high and prolonged doses* it is a stupefacient, slowing down the circulation, entailing muscular paresis, cerebral congestion and the problems of *chronic absinthism* (Cadéac and Meunier)

Indications:
Internal use:
- *nervous dyspepsia, flatulence, aerophagy* and vomiting of nervous origin
- nauseous migraine, vertigo
- painful menstrual periods
- infantile colic
- cardiovascular erethism *(false angina pectoris,* palpitations)

– cardiac fatigue
– *asthma,* bronchial spasm, cough, difficulty in breathing
– lacteal insufficiency
– impotence, frigidity (?)
– oliguria

External use:
 – used in dentifrices

Methods of use:
 – infusion: 1 teaspoon to a cup of boiling water; take one cupful after meals.
 – powder: 0.20 to 2g per day, in the form of tablets.
 – tincture: 1 to 3g per day (1g = 20 drops); 10 to 20 drops for children.
 – spirit: 5 to 15g (contains 2g of essence to 98g of alcohol at 90°).
 – syrup: 30 to 60g (children): 1 teaspoonful at a time.
 – *balm of anisated sulphur* (bronchial conditions):

sulphur...	1g
essence of aniseed.................................	4g

6 to 8 drops in a potion.

 – *antispasmodic potion:*

essence of aniseed...........................	10 drops
sulphuric ether	20 drops
laudanum (Sydenham's)	12 drops
syrup of poppies	50g
infusion of Chinese aniseed......................	150g

 – *liqueur of aniseed:*

crushed seeds of aniseed	40g
cinnamon.......................................	1g
sugar...	500g
spirits	1 litre

leave to macerate for six weeks; filter; take a liqueur glass after meals (digestive, carminative).
– see under *Cinnamon* for aromatic tincture of arnica (contusions).

N.B.
The seeds of aniseed, together with those of caraway, coriander and fennel, used in equal parts, make up the carminative mixture of the "four warming seeds".

Basil

Sweet or Common Basil

Ocimum basilicum

Labiatae

There are about a hundred and fifty varieties of basil, differing for instance in the shape of the leaves or their size or colour – one type nettle-leaved, another like lettuce. Originally coming from Asia, basil is found in both northern and southern hemispheres.

Parts used: flowering tops and the essence obtained by steam distillation of the leaves.

Principal known constitutents: essential oil: ocimen, linalol, estragol.

Properties:
- restorative, stimulant, *tonic* (especially of the nerves: Bodart. Also of adrenal cortex)
- *antispasmodic* (first stimulates, then lessens cerebro-spinal activity: Cadéac and Meunier); calmative
- stomachic
- intestinal antiseptic
- emmenagogue

Indications:
Internal use:
- *nervous debility* (mental fatigue)
- anxiety
- *nervous insomnia*, vertigo
- *gastric spasm*, dyspepsia
- intestinal infections
- whooping cough
- *migraine*
- *epilepsy* (Pliny)
- *paralysis*
- *gout*
- scanty menstrual periods

External use:
- loss of the sense of smell due to chronic nasal catarrh, rhinitis
- wasp stings, snake bites (first-aid treatment)

Methods of Use:
Internal:
- infusion: one dessertspoonful in a cup of boiling water. Take one cupful after every meal (digestive).
- essence: 2 to 5 drops three times a day in an alcoholic solution, or in honey.
- *antispasmodic syrup:*

```
essence of basil ..................................  1g
essence of marjoram.............................  1g
powdered sugar...................................  50g
```

½ to 1 teaspoon in a cup of lime-blossom or verbena tea after meals.

External
- powdered dried leaves: sternutatory (i.e. causing sneezing); use to treat *loss of the sense of smell* due to chronic rhinitis, nasal catarrh.
- essence or bruised leaves: rub on wasp stings and snake bites (first-aid treatment).

N.B.
Basil may be used instead of thyme as a condiment; it is a good addition to soup and salad which it asepticises – and of course it is used in stuffing for duck and in the famous *Soupe au pistou*, one of the most celebrated dishes from Provence.

Soupe au pistou (quantities to serve four)

250g tomatoes	6 carrots
2 or 3 potatoes	100g haricot beans
100g green beans	celery
1 large onion	a handful of basil
2 cloves of garlic	150g grated cheese
1 cup oil	

Heat 2 tablespoons of oil in a saucepan, fry the onion, add the tomatoes cut in quarters, cover and cook gently for a few minutes. Add 1½ litres water and bring to the boil. Add the haricot beans, cook for 30 minutes, then add the other vegetables (diced). Season and cook for a further 15 minutes. Meanwhile, have prepared a paste of basil and garlic crushed in a mortar with the remainder of the oil. Put the paste in a soup tureen, pour the soup over it and sprinkle with grated cheese.

Bergamot

Citrus bergamia

Rutaceae

A variety of citrus.

Parts used: the essence, obtained by expressing the outer part of the peel of the freshly picked fruit. 100 kilos of fruit yield approximately 500g of essence. The pulp is used in making citric acid.

Principal known constituents: essence; linalyl acetate (35 to 45%), limonene, linalol.

Properties:
- *antiseptic* (intestinal)
- *antispasmodic*, calmative
- stomachic
- *vermifuge*

Indications:
- Loss of appetite
- *colic* and *intestinal infection*
- dyspepsia, painful digestion
- *intestinal parasites*

Method of use:
- essence: 1–6 drops per day

N.B.
Apart from its pharmaceutical use, the essence of bergamot is widely used in the perfume and confectionery industries.

Borneol (Borneo Camphor)

Borneol is obtained from a tree growing naturally in Borneo and Sumatra, the *Dryobalanops camphora*. It is the mature tree which produces borneol, which exudes naturally under the bark where it is found in crystallised masses of varying sizes; the young tree produces only a clear yellow liquid – "liquid camphor".

Principal known constituents: it is an alcohol, and may thus be distinguished from Japanese camphor (the camphor commonly in use) which is a ketone.

Borneol, which was known long before camphor, has always been regarded as a panacea. For many hundreds of years it was considered a powerful remedy against the plague; its therapeutic reputation was such that King Chrosroes II of Persia preserved it among the treasures of his palace in Babylon. Writers down the centuries have proclaimed its virtues. In Italy, a fairly recent archaeological find allowed the identification of organic matter perfectly preserved for over 2,000 years in a jar of borneol. Borneo camphor has always enjoyed a very high reputation in India and China.

Properties:
Internal and external use:
– *powerful antiseptic*
– general and cardiac *tonic*
– *stimulant of the adrenal cortex*
– desensitising agent

Indications:
– *depressive states*, convalescence
– *infectious diseases*

Methods of use:
– in association with other essences (0.25 to 0.50%); it may be ingested or, in dilute form, given intramuscularly.
– it is also given in the form of various ethers such as isovalerianate of bornyl in capsules or *perles* of 0.25ctg, at a dosage of 3 to 5 a day, as a *sedative* similar in action to valerian.

N.B.
Numerous essences obtained from European plants also contain borneol, for instance hyssop and rosemary.

Cajuput

Melaleuca leucodendron

Myrtaceae

A tree which grows abundantly in the Philippines, Malaysia, the Moluccas and Celébes.

Parts used: the essence, obtained by steam distillation of the leaves and buds.

Principal known constituents: cineol (60 to 75%), d-pinene, terpineol, aldehydes.

Properties:
Internal use:
− *general antiseptic* (pulmonary, intestinal, urinary)
− antispasmodic, antineuralgic, calmative
− vermifuge

External use:
− antiseptic
− analgesic
− cicatrising

Indications:
Internal use:
− enteritis, dysentery
− cystitis, urethritis
− chronic pulmonary diseases (bronchitis, tuberculosis)
− chronic laryngitis and pharyngitis
− gastric spasm
− asthma
− nervous vomiting
− painful periods
− rheumatism, gout
− hysteria, epilepsy
− intestinal parasites

External use:
− toothache and earache
− chronic laryngitis
− rheumatic neuralgia
− sores
− dermatoses (skin diseases) − psoriasis, acne, etc.

Methods of use:

Internal:
- essence: 2 to 5 drops in honey water 3 to 4 times a day (or in an alcoholic solution).

External:
- the essence in inhalations (laryngitis).
- ointments at one-fifth or one-tenth, or alcoholic solution, in friction rubs for rheumatic neuralgia, and abdominal friction rubs as a vermifuge; also applied on skin diseases and sores.
- for toothache: 1 drop of essence on the decayed tooth.
- for earache: a little piece of cottonwool soaked in the essence and placed in the ear.

Roman Camomile

Anthemis nobilis

Compositae

Also known as Sweet Camomile, Chamomile.

Parts used: flowers, the whole plant, essence obtained by steam distillation of the flowers.

Principal known constituents: essence (angelic and isobutyric ethers, a bitter principal, a special camphor, anthemene, sesquiterpenes: azulene, artemol), resin, gum phytosterol, calcium, sulphur.

Properties (used since ancient times):
  Internal use:
  – tonic
  – *antispasmodic*, calmative
  – analgesic
  – mild nerve sedative (children)
  – apéritif
  – stimulant (increases production of white blood corpuscles)
  – *stomachic*, digestive stimulant
  – *antianaemic*
  – *vermifuge*
  – *emmenagogue*
  – vulnerary (ulceration or irritation of the intestine)
  – bactericide (bacteriostatic)
  – febrifuge
  – sudorific
  – cholagogue
  – hypnotic

  External use:
  – antineuralgic (rheumatism, gout)
  – *antiophthalmic*
  – *antiphlogistic* and healing (Eichholz)

Indications:
  Internal use:
  – *migraine*
  – neuralgia (especially *facial neuralgia*: Lecointe, H. Leclerc)
  – painful teething in children
  – vertigo
  – problems associated with the menopause
  – insomnia

- *loss of appetite*
- *dyspepsia*, painful or *difficult digestion*, flatulence
- gastric and intestinal ulcers
- digestive problems in children (diarrhoea, gastric and intestinal cramp)
- infantile diseases
- enteritis
- *anaemia*
- congestion of spleen and liver
- *nervous depression*, hysterics, nervous crisis
- irritability
- convulsions
- *menstrual problems (dysmenorrhoea, amenorrhoea)* linked to nervous troubles
- lumbar pains and headaches during *influenza* (H. Leclerc)
- intestinal parasites (Ascaris, Oxyuris)
- *intermittent fevers, fevers of nervous origin*

External use:
- *conjunctivitis*, inflammation of the eyelids, ophthalmia
- inflamed skin conditions
- burns, boils, herpes, eczema
- sores, wounds (minor and infected)
- vulvar pruritis, urticaria
- rheumatic pains and gout

Methods of use:
Internal:
- infusion: 5 to 10 *flowerheads* per cup, Take one cupful *before* meals (Alimat): *loss of appetite.*
- *powder: in honey, 2 to 10g per day.*
- *essence: 2 to 4 drops, 2 or 3 times a day (in honey water or in an alcoholic solution).*
- as a vermifuge: 1 tablespoonful of chopped plant per cup; boil and infuse for 10 minutes. Take one cup first thing in the morning and a cupful half an hour before meals.

External:
- for *conjunctivitis* and *inflammation of the eyelids:* 1 tablespoonful of flowers per cup; boil and infuse for 10 minutes. Use when washing or with an eye-bath.
- for *rheumatic pains and gout, oil of camomile:*

  dried flowers 20g
  olive oil 100g

  Heat in a bain-marie for 2 hours, strain with pressure and filter through fine muslin cloth; add 10g of camphor. Use for friction rubs.
- a decoction for used in the *bath* or in *compresses* or washes in the treatment of dermatoses, burns, boils, herpes, eczema. It has *antiphlogistic*, relaxing and deodorant properties.

German Camomile

Matricaria chamomilla

Compositae

Also known as Common Camomile, Wild Chamomile.

This plant yields the oil of camomile which is used externally.

Parts used: flowers, seeds.

Principal known constituents: essence containing ethers of caprylic and monylic acid, a hydrocarbon and *azulene* (see Note 1).

Properties:
Internal use:
— antispasmodic, calmative
— *analgesic*
— *stimulant*
— sudorific
— febrifuge
— cholagogue
— bactericide
— *vermifuge* (Ascaris, Oxyuris)
— *emmenagogue* (Gibbs and Brow)
— mild nerve sedative (children)
— stimulant of leucocyte production (ingestion triples the number of white blood corpuscles: Dady)

External use:
— antiphlogistic and healing (Eichholz)

Indications are the same as for English Camomile.

Methods of use:
Internal:
— infusion: a tablespoonful to a cup of boiling water; infuse for 10 minutes (or 1 hour according to Leclerc), strain. Take 1 cupful between meals (it is very bitter).
— powder: 2 to 5g per day in tablets: "fresh powder of the flowers of *Anthemis nobilis* or *Martricaria chamomilla*" triturated (i.e. ground) with a desired quantity of sugar, 4g. Enough for 6 tablets which should be taken in 24 hours (Leclerc), between meals.
— "mother tincture": adults, 10 drops on a sugar lump after meals; children, 2 to 3 drops in a little water or milk twice a day.

– suppositories and enemas: 0.75g to 1g of powder (non-irritant).

External – see English Camomile.

N.B.
1. Azulene is a fatty substance discovered in the essence of *Matricaria* (camazulene). It possesses healing and antiphlogistic properties which have been studied chiefly by the Germans, and in France by Caujolle. Numerous experiments have shown its remarkable effectiveness in treating various inflammations of the skin, eczema, leg ulcers, vulvar pruritis, urticaria, and also chronic gastritis, colitis, cystitis and certain kinds of asthma.

   The bacteriostatic effect of azulene is produced at a concentration of 1 part in 2,000 against Staphylococcus aureus, haemolytic Streptococcus and Proteus vulgaris in particular. Infected wounds have been healed using concentrations of from 1 part in 85,000 to 1 part in 170,000.

   Manufacturers of all kinds of creams, lotions and soaps are increasingly using azulene in their products.
2. An infusion of camomile was formerly used as an after-shampoo rinse to counter loss of hair. Nowadays it is rarely used except, because of its secondary action, as a bleach. In this case at least, however, fashion is on the right track, for it is in accord with aesthetic and hygienic practice as well as being therapeutically sound.

Caraway

Carum carvi

Umbelliferae

Caraway is grown in Germany, the Low Countries, Scandinavia and Siberia.

Parts used: seeds, essence obtained by steam distillation of the crushed fruit.

Principal known constituents: essence (carvone, 45–60%; carvene, 30%).

Properties: (compare with those of aniseed):
Internal use:
− *stimulant* (circulatory and cardiac)
− stomachic, digestive stimulant
− apéritif
− *antispasmodic*
− *carminative*
− diuretic
− *vermifuge*
− emmenagogue
− galactagogue (?)

External use:
− parasiticide

Indications:
Internal use:
− loss of appetite
− indigestion, *nervous dyspepsia*
− *gastric and intestinal spasm*
− *aerophagy*
− flatulence, distension of the stomach
− putrefactive fermentations
− cardiovascular erethism (false angina pectoris, palpitations)
− intestinal parasites
− vertigo
− difficult menstrual periods
− lacteal insufficiency (?)

External use:
- scabies
− mange (in dogs)
− used in toothpaste

Methods of use:
- infusion: 1 teaspoonful of *seeds* to a cup of boiling water; infuse for 10 minutes. Take 1 cupful after each meal. Leclerc suggests the addition of 1 teaspoonful of oleo-saccharum of caraway at a strength of one-twentieth.
- essence: 1 to 3 drops in honey water or in an alcoholic solution 2 or 3 times a day.
- *spirits of caraway:*

alcohol	1 litre
caraway seeds	40g
sugar	200g

leave to macerate for 8–10 days, then decant. Take a liquer-glassful after meals.

N.B.
1. Caraway is a much-used condiment in Germany and Arab countries as well as England, in pastries, sauces, sausage, sauerkraut and bread. It is also used in the making of certain liqueurs (Kümmel).
2. Gemeiner suggested the following formula in 1907 for the treatment of demodetic mange in dogs:

essence of caraway	10g
alcohol	10g
castor oil	150g

Paint the affected parts.

Cinnamon

Cinnamomum zeylanicum

Lauraceae

Cinnamon of Ceylon, the best-known variety of cinnamon, comes from the Sri Lankan cinnamon tree (*Cinnamomum zelanicum*), an evergreen native to Sri Lanka, the East Indies, the Antilles, Java and Madagascar. The inner bark of the new shoots is the part used, and this is gathered every two years. The fragments of bark are dried and formed into the little sticks which are sold commercially.

Chinese cinnamon (which is less sought after) comes from the *Cinnamomum cassia*, a tree found in Annam and southern China. Its powder has a redder colour.

Parts used: the bark and the essence obtained by steam distillation of bark and leaves.

Principal known constituents: the essential oil from the bark contains 65–75% cinnamic aldehyde, 4–10% eugenol, carbides, terpenic alcohols. I-pinene, cineol, phellandrene, furfurol, cymene, linalol, sugar, mucilage, tannin, starch, mannite.

The essence from the leaves contains 70–75% eugenol, only 3% cinnamic aldehyde, benzyl benzoate, linalol, safrol.

Properties:
Internal use:
- *stimulant* (circulatory, cardiac and respiratory)
- stomachic, digestive stimulant
- *antiseptic,* antiputrefactive *(Cinnamomum zeylanicum* kills Eberth's bacillus (typhoid) at a dose of 1 part in 300)
- carminative
- *vermifuge*
- *antispasmodic*
- haemostatic
- lightly astringent
- aphrodisiac (mild)
- emmenagogue (it has sometimes been considered abortifacient)
- slightly raises body temperature, stimulating production of saliva, tears and mucus

External use:
- parasiticide

Indications:

Internal use:
- general debility
- the aching produced by fever; influenza; conditions resulting from chill
- *influenzal debility*
- fainting, difficulty in breathing
- contagious diseases
- intestinal infections (cholera, typhoid fever)
- gastric atony, sluggish digestion, atonic dyspepsia
- intestinal parasites
- *digestive spasm*, colitis, gastralgia
- diarrhoea
- metrorrhagia, leucorrhoea
- haemoptysis
- impotence
- scanty menstrual periods
- it was formerly given to the melancholic, to people with digestive problems and to old people during the winter months

External use:
- lice, scabies
- wasp stings, snake bites
- contusions, toothache (aromatic tincture of arnica)
- care of teeth (q.v. *Clove*)

Methods of use:

Internal:
- infusion, of the bark: 8 to 15g to 1 litre of water
- *powder:* 0.50 to 2g a day in tablets
- *distilled cinnamon water:* 10 to 50g in syrups and draughts
- *20% tincture:* 1.50 to 10g in syrups and draughts
- hot sweet wine and cinnamon for *chills* or aching from fever and for *influenza*
- *essence:* 2 to 3 drops in honey water twice a day
    for *influenza:* 5–10 drops every 2 hours
    for *cholera:* 5 to 10 drops every half hour
- a mixture for *dyspepsia:*

    blackcurrant leaves 10g
    cinnamon of Ceylon............................... 1g
    clove... 1g

in an infusion, to 1 litre of water. Take 1 cupful after meals.

– a draught to be taken for *metrorrhagia:*

> tincture of cinnamon 25g
> cinnamon water 150g
> acetic ether 5g
> syrup of the peel of bitter orange 30g

to be taken in a 24-hour period.

External:
– may be mixed with other essences and used as an *inhalation* (for conditions of the respiratory tract)
– for *lice* and *scabies:*

> essence of cinnamon ....
> essence of thyme.................................
> essence of rosemary .... } 2.50g of each
> essence of pine..................................
> a solution of sulphoricinate of soda at 30% 90g

– *for scabies,* see also under *Lavender,* Helmerich's ointment.
– put the essence on wasp stings and snake bites (first-aid treatment).

N.B.
1. Cinnamon is one of the constituents of compound spirit of lemon balm, Garus's elixir, Todd's potion, etc; it is also used in cough lozenges and dentifrices.

1 – *Cordial potion (Codex)*

> tincture of cinnamon 10g
> Banyuls 150g
> syrup... 40g

2 – *Compound Cinnamon wine* (recipe of the Hôpitaux de Paris): *cordial*

> red wine.. 100g
> tincture of cinnamon 8g
> spirit of balm.................................... 6g
> simple syrup 30g

(this formula is similar to that of the Hôpitaux Militaires of 1821).

3 – *Aromatic tincture of arnica:*

> flowers of arnica 50g
>
> clove... 10g
> cinnamon....................................... 10g
> ginger 10g
> aniseed... 100g
> alcohol .... 1 litre

leave to macerate for 8 days and strain.

A spoonful in half a glass of sugared water, 2 or 3 times a day, in the case of *falls* and *contusion*; it is a good *antiodontalgic* (toothache).

4 – *Chaussier's antiseptic elixir:*

quinquina	64g
cascarilla	16g
saffron	2g
Spanish wine	500g
cinnamon	12g
spirits (brandy)	500g

leave for several days, strain and add:

sugar	150g
sulphuric ether	6g

use in the treatment of typhus (this preparation was used in 1814–15).

5 – *Italian essence:*

cinnamon	90g
greater cardamom	60g
galingale	60g
clove	15g
long pepper	12g
nutmeg	8g
ambergris	0.2g
musk	0.2g
alcohol at 90°	1 litre

leave to blend. Filter.
Aphrodisiac: 20 to 30 drops on a sugar lump.

6 – *Aphrodisiac wine:*

vanilla beans	30g
cinnamon	30g
ginseng	30g
rhubarb	30g
Malaga wine	1 litre
or mature Chablis	

leave to macerate for 15 days in the wine, shaking daily. Filter and add 15 drops of tincture of amber.

7 – *Liqueur known as "Parfait amour":*

zest of lemon	40g
thyme	30g
cinnamon	15g
vanilla	10g
coriander	10g
mace	10g
spirits	2 litres

leave to macerate for 15 days and add sugar-water made with 2 kg sugar to a litre of water. Mix the two together and filter.

2. See under *Clove* for two formulae for dentifrices and an aromatic vinegar. See under *Hyssop* for the formula for the herbal elixir of Grande Chartreuse.

3. Cinnamon used to be regarded as a rare and precious substance. Those who could obtain it used it in Hippocras (a tonic drink made of sugared wine in which cinnamon, ginger and cloves have been infused), pastries and sweetmeats. Many pharmaceutical preparations contained cinnamon, and it was also used as incense and as a perfume.

4. A recipe for a snack, passed on by Leclerc: sprinkle cinnamon on hot buttered toast.

5. In the past people used to wear little boxes filled with aromatic herbs – one of which was cinnamon – to ward off contagious diseases. According to Chamberland, writing in 1887, three essences "possess the greatest antiseptic power, whether through their vapours or when used in solution: these are those of cinnamon from Ceylon, Chinese cinnamon and origanum".

6. Here is a formula which always seems effective against *colds* and *influenza*, as long as it is taken as soon as the first symptoms appear. Most people will find this "remedy", which can be made from everyday ingredients, pleasant to take:

> a tot of whisky, to which is added half a squeezed lemon, a tablespoonful of honey and a large glass of hot water in which a small piece of cinnamon and a clove have been boiled for 2 to 3 minutes. Leave to infuse for 20 minutes.

Clove

Eugenia caryophyllata

Myrtaceae

The clove tree is a small evergreen with light grey leaves and a smooth bark, growing in the Moluccas, Réunion, the Antilles and Madagascar.

Parts used: the flower buds ("cloves") and the essence extracted from the buds, which are allowed to dry naturally, by steam distillation. The extracted essence constitutes 16–20%, by weight, of the cloves.

Production: 10,000 tonnes of cloves per annum from Zanzibar and Pemba Island ($\frac{7}{8}$ of world production), and 1,000 tonnes from Madagascar. One tree yields an average of 7–10 kg of cloves a year.

Principal known constituents: gum, tannin, caryophyline, essential oil: 70–85% eugenol, aceteugenol, methyl alcohol, methyl salicylate, furfurol, pinene, vanillin, caryophyllene.

Properties:
Internal use:
- stimulant (general and mental)
- *powerful antiseptic* (see Notes): a 1% emulsion of clove has an antiseptic strength 3 to 4 times greater than that of phenol
- stomachic and carminative
- antineuralgic
- caustic
- antispasmodic
- vermifuge
- uterine tonic (during labour)
- aphrodisiac (?)
- anticancer (?)
External use:
- parasiticide
- antiseptic
- cicatrising
- analgesic
- caustic

Indications:
Internal use:
- physical and mental debility (memory deficiency)
- prevention of contagious and infectious diseases (formerly used against the plague)
- dyspepsia, diarrhoea, intestinal spasm
- flatulence
- pulmonary infections, tuberculosis

114

- toothache
- intestinal parasites
- preparation for childbirth
- malignant conditions (?)
- impotence (?)
- formerly recommended for headaches, deafness, dropsy and gout

External use:
- scabies
- sores, infected wounds, leg ulcers
- toothache
- corneal leucoma
- lupus
- mosquito and clothes-moth repellent

Methods of use:
Internal:
- 2 to 4 drops of the *essence* 3 times a day in an alcoholic solution, or in honey water.
- *preparation for childbirth:* use cloves in soups during the last few months of pregnancy, and take an infusion of cloves before the onset of labour.
- *Neapolitan aphrodisiac pastilles:*

sugar	500 parts
mastic	12 parts
saffron	8 parts
musk	1 part
ginger	2 parts
clove	2 parts
ambergris	4 parts
infusion of catnip	as desired

Make pastilles weighing 0.5 to 1g each. Take 4 to 5 a day.
- use cloves in everyday *cooking* (soups, stews, marinades).

External:
- in fumigations.
- in lotions, compresses and mouthwashes (a solution of the essence or an infusion of cloves).
- 80 years ago, W. A. Briggs used the antiseptic properties of essence of clove to disinfect operating theatres and the hands of surgeons, obstetricians and nurses. With the aid of this essence he treated simple, contused and infected wounds as well as leg ulcers. In treating abscesses he plugged the cavities with gauze moistened with neat or diluted essence. Leclerc recommends essence of clove as an excellent dressing for the umbilical cord since it is neither toxic nor irritant and is, to a certain degree, analgesic.

- a Russian doctor has used aqueous extract of clove in the treatment of corneal leucomas after the inflammation has subsided, the instillations clearing the specks by reabsorbing the infiltrates and improving the nutrition of the scar tissue of the cornea.
- in friction rubs to treat *lupus*, use in an alcoholic solution at a strength of 5–10%.
- to treat *scabies*, see under *Lavender* (Helmerich's ointment).
- to repel mosquitos and moths, use an orange stuck with cloves.

N.B.

1. The Moluccas were swept by several previously unknown epidemics after the Dutch destroyed all the clove trees in Ternate. In the old days, oranges stuck with cloves were in common use as a protection against contagion.

2. *Eugenol* is increasingly taking the place of essence of clove as
   - an antithermic
   - an *antiseptic* (for pulmonary tuberculosis: 0.80ctg a day in capsule form)
   - a disinfectant and cauterising agent in dental surgery.

3. Clove *essence* is one of the ingredients of *Koheul*, an ophthalmic ointment used by the Arabs.

4. An *infusion of cloves* together with boric acid and glycerine makes an antiseptic liquid used in the preservation of meat. (One single clove added to boiled beef will preserve it for 24 hours).

5. *Formulae for aromatic dentifrices:*

   a)

essence of cinnamon	1g
essence of Chinese aniseed	2g
essence of clove	2g
essence of mint	8g
tincture of benzoin	8g
tincture of cochineal	20g
tincture of guaiacum	8g
tincture of pyrethrum	8g
alcohol (80°)	1 litre

   Mix all the ingredients. Filter after 24 hours. Take ½ teaspoonful in a glass of warm water.

   b)

cinnamon essence	1g
essence of aniseed	2g
essence of clove	3g
essence of mint	8g
tincture of benzoin	5g
ground cochineal	5g
alcohol (80°)	1 litre

6. *English aromatic vinegar* (smelling salts):

acetic acid (solid)	250g
camphor	60g
essential oil of lavender	0.50g
essential oil of clove	2g
essential oil of cinnamon	1g

7. See *Rosemary* for a formula for an aphrodisiac bath.
   See *Cinnamon* for the composition of *aromatic tincture of arnica, Italian essence* and a dyspepsia mixture. See also the formula for anti-flu toddy (Note 6).
   See Chapter 6 for "Vinegar of the Four Thieves" (Marseilles vinegar).

8. The West Germans recently developed a clove-based general anaesthetic. This drug does away with "premeds" and allows the patient to regain consciousness 15 to 20 minutes after the anaesthetic. (According to Cadéac and Meunier, clove essence is endowed with opiate properties; Sydenham's laudanum contains clove essence as an adjuvant to opium).

9. Clove was for a long time the most expensive of the spices; it was regarded as a panacea for centuries. It could be used much more widely in medicine than it is today. But it is an ingredient of many drinks and liqueurs, e.g. raspail, cherry brandy and ambrosia.

10. Essence of clove is otherwise used in perfumery and in the manufacture of printing inks, glues and varnish.

Coriander

Coriandrum sativum

Umbelliferae

The coriander plant is found in Central Europe and the Soviet Union. It is distinguished by its ability to become acclimatised in temperate countries; the Egyptians first introduced it to Europe, and in the 18th century it was cultivated in the region of Paris.

Parts used: fruit (improperly called seed), essence obtained by steam distillation of ground seeds (yield 1%).

Principal known constituents: essence: 90% of coriandrol (isomer of borneol), geraniol, pinene, cineol, terpinene, etc.

Properties (analogous to those of aniseed and caraway):
Internal use:
 – *carminative*
 – *stomachic*
 – stimulant
 – formerly held to be an aphrodisiac and to aid the memory

External use:
 – analgesic

Indications (q.v. aniseed and caraway):
Internal use:
 – *dyspepsia, painful digestion, nervous dyspepsia*
 – *flatulence, aerophagy*
 – *spasm*
 – anorexia nervosa (loss of appetite)
 – nervous debility

External use:
 – rheumatic pains

Methods of use:
Internal:
 – *infusion:* 1 teaspoonful of seeds to a cup of water. Boil and infuse for 10 minutes. Drink 1 cupful after each meal.
 – *tincture:* 10 to 20 drops after meals.
 – *essence:* 1 to 3 drops in honey water 2 to 3 times a day after meals.

External:
 – in lotions and ointments for *rheumatic pain.*

N.B.
1. The fresh fruit, the size of a grain of pepper, is foul-smelling. it becomes pleasant and aromatic when desiccated.
2. The juice of *freshly-picked* plants when ingested in weak doses has properties similar to those of alcohol: it excites and then depresses. Larger doses lead to manic drunkenness and eventual prostration (Cadéac and Meunier).
3. Coriander is used as a seasoning; it is also used in brewing to flavour beer. The Algerians use a mixture of coriander, pepper and salt to preserve meat.
4. Many apéritifs and liqueurs contain coriander, e.g. the Basque drink *izzara*, ambrosia, and ratafia (together with angelica, celery and fennel); it is also found in brandy, in Senna syrup and in Melissa cordial. It is an indispensable seasoning for dishes prepared "à la Grecque" – mushrooms, artichokes, etc.
5. The famous toilet water first produced by the Carmelites in Paris in the 17th century owes much of its success to coriander.

Cypress

Cupressus sempervirens

Coniferae

Cypress is traditionally a tree of graveyards. But it has many other qualities . . . Paul Vasseur described it as "an exclamation-mark on a happy landscape". *C. sempervirens* is the cypress of southern Europe, also known as Italian cypress.

Parts used: cones, leaves, shoots, essential oil obtained by distillation of leaves and fruit ("cypress nuts"). This tree has been used since antiquity (e.g. by the Assyrians, also by Hippocrates).

Compare: Witch hazel (Hamamelis), hydrastis, horse chestnut, cotton plant, viburnum.

Principal known constituents: tannins analogous to those of the bark and leaves of Hamamelis; an *essential oil:* d-pinene, d-campene, d-sylvestrene, cymene, a ketone, sabinol, a terpenic alcohol, valeric acid, camphor of cypress.

Properties:
Internal use:
- astringent
- *vasoconstrictor*, venous tonic (superior to Hamamelis, according to Leclerc)
- *antispasmodic*
- antisudorific
- *antirheumatic*, diuretic
- general *restorative* (in particular of the *nervous system*)
- anticancer (?)

External use:
- vasoconstrictor
- deodorant (of the feet)

Indications:
Internal use:
- haemoptysis (spitting blood)
- *haemorrhoids, varicose veins*
- *ovarian disorders* (dysmenorrhoea, *metorrhagia*)
- menopause
- *whooping cough*, spasmodic cough
- *enuresis* (C. Barbin)

120

- *influenza*
- aphonia (loss of voice)
- rheumatism
- *irritability*, spasm
- malignant conditions (?)

External use:
- haemorrhoids
- excessive sweating of the feet

Methods of use:
Internal:
- *fluid extract* and tincture: 15 to 30 drops before the two main meals *(enuresis)*; 30 to 60 drops for other indications.
- *tincture* of cypress, like that of Hamamelis, is given for haemorrhoids, varicose veins, metorrhagia, menopausal problems, haemoptysis (Leclerc): 30 to 60 drops before the two main meals.
- soft extract: 0.15 to 0.20g per day in pills.
- the wood is used chiefly as a sudorific and diuretic.
- *essential oil:* 2 to 4 drops in honey water 2 or 3 times a day (or in an alcoholic solution).

External:
- aqueous solution (at 5%) of tincture or of fluid extract as an enema.
- decoction of 20 to 30g to 1 litre of water in foot baths for offensively smelling feet.
- suppositories: 0.15 to 0.30g soft extract.
- *essential oil:* a few drops on the pillow 4 or 5 times a day in cases of whooping and spasmodic cough.
- *anti-haemorrhoidal suppository:*

soft extract of cypress nuts	0.15g
soft extract of opium	2cg
soft extract of belladonna	2cg
cocoa-butter	5g

for a suppository: 1 to 3 per day (Leclerc).
- *ointment for haemorrhoids:*

soft extract of cypress	1g
balm of poplar	50g

N.B.
An infusion of the globular cone of the cypress has cicatrising properties in the treatment of wounds.

Eucalyptus

Eucalyptus globulus

Myrtaceae

Also known as Gum-tree.
More than 300 varieties are known, of which about 50 may be found on the shores of the Mediterranean.

Origin: Australia, Tasmania. It is now found throughout Europe and North Africa. It is used in infusions (leaves, flowerbuds) and inhalations (leaves, essential oil); it is also taken orally in the form of essential oil, usually in association with other essences. The essence is extracted from the leaves by steam distillation.

Principal known constituents: tannins, essence consisting of eucalyptol (80–85%), phellandrene, aromadendrene, eudesmol, pinene, camphene, valeric, butyric and caproic aldehydes, ethyl and amyl alcohols.

Long experience has demonstrated the effects of eucalyptol, an excellent pulmonary antiseptic which is partially eliminated through bronchial secretion. In fact the effect produced by the other components of eucalyptus essence is even greater. The essence has a bactericidal power stronger than that of pure eucalyptol, as Cuthbert Hall has shown in his experiments on various microbial cultures *(on Eucalyptus oils, especially in relation to their bactericidal power*, Schimmel, Bulletin, October 1904). This is probably due to the presence of a small quantity of ozone, produced by the oxidation of the phellandrenes and aromadendrenes.

Properties:
Internal use:
– *general antiseptic*, in particular of the *respiratory* and urinary tracts
– *balsamic* (soothes coughs, expectorant)
– *hypoglycaemic* (Faulds, Trabut)
– antirheumatic, antineuralgic
– febrifuge
– *vermifuge*
– stimulant

External use:
– bactericide (used in a spray, an emulsion of 2% essence of eucalyptus kills 70% of ambient Staphylococci)
– parasiticide
– preventive of contagious and pulmonary diseases
– insect repellent (mosquitos, gnats)

Indications:

Internal use:

- *conditions of the respiratory tract:* acute and chronic *bronchitis, influenza, pulmonary tuberculosis,* pulmonary gangrene, asthma, cough, pneumonia
- conditions of the urinary tract: various infections, *colibacillosis,* cystitis
- *diabetes*
- various diseases and fevers: malaria, typhus, measles, scarlet fever, cholera (prophylactic against measles and scarlet fever: Milne's method (see Note 1))
- *rheumatism,* neuralgia
- *intestinal parasites:* Ascaris, Oxyuris
- *migraine*
- *debility*

External use:

- wounds, burns: used on dressings aids formation of new tissue
- pulmonary conditions, influenza
- sinusitis
- lice (Sergent and Holey)
- mosquito repellent

Methods of use:

Internal:

- *infusion:* 3 to 4 leaves (or 1 tablespoonful of chopped leaves) per cupful. Boil for 1 minute and infuse for 10. Take 3 to 5 cups per day.
- powdered leaves: tablets of 0.50g, 6 to 10 a day.
- alcoholic tincture: 2 to 4g a day in a draught (children: 5 drops for each year of age per day).
- tincture at 20%: 1 to 10g a day in draughts.
- syrup: 30 to 100g a day (20g = 0.70g for eucalyptus leaves).
- *essential oil:* may be used either in drops (2 to 5 drops, 2 or 3 times a day in honey water, usually with other essences – 20 drops to the gram, maximum daily dose 2 to 3g) or in the form of *perles* or capsules of from 0.10 to 0.20g (0.20 to 2g per day).

External:

- infusion: to fumigate rooms, or in inhalations (10g per litre).
- the essence in inhalations (10 to 15 drops in a bowl of boiling water).
- *formula for inhalations* (influenza, sinusitis, bronchitis)

essential oil of lavender	1g
essential oil of pine (needles)	2g
essential oil of thyme	2g
essential oil of eucalyptus	4g
90° alcohol	150cc

123

1 dessertspoonful to 1 tablespoonful in a bowl of boiling water. For 2 to 3 inhalations a day for 8 to 15 days.
— *tablets for inhalation:*

menthol	0.001g
essence of eucalyptus	0.06g
essence of thyme	0.03g
tincture of benzoin	0.03g

for one tablet. 1 or 2 tablets added to a bowl of very hot water.
— wounds: infusion, diluted essence.
— *burns:*
oily antiseptic mixture (Hôpital Broussais):

essences of eucalyptus and thyme	2g each
essences of rosemary and lavender	3g each
menthol	0.50g
methyl salicylate	1g
"baume Tranquille"	100g
poppyseed oil	1,000g

for dressings.
— *disinfectant mixture:*

essence of eucalyptus	15g
phenol	15g
essence of turpentine	100g

leave to evaporate in the room (e.g. on compresses).
— *lotion to repel mosquitos, gnats:*

essence of eucalyptus	56g
essence of citronella	56g
saturated alcoholic solution of phenic acid	6 drops

paint on to the skin.
— another lotion:

essence of citronella	26g
essence of cedar	28g
camphorated alcohol	26g

paint on to exposed parts.

N.B.
1. *Milne's method:* a method of treating eruptive fevers, particularly measles and scarlet fever, by which contagion is prevented without the need to isolate the patient. This consists in repeatedly painting the tonsils and pharynx with 10% carbolated oil, applying an ointment of pure eucalyptus essence to the skin, and protecting the patient's head, for as long as he continues to cough and sneeze, with a veil (attached to a hoop around the head) which is regularly sprinkled with eucalyptus essence.
2. A variety of eucalyptus *(Eucalyptus coccifera,* var. Favieri) is resistant to frost.

Fennel

Foeniculum vulgare

Umbelliferae

There are two varieties of fennel, sweet fennel *(F. vulgare)*, and Florence fennel *(F. vulgare dulce)* which may be enjoyed as a vegetable in the manner of celery.

Fennel is grown in the Mediterranean region, Central Europe, India, Japan, Asia and America.

Parts used: roots, seeds, leaves, essence obtained by steam distillation of the pulverised seeds.

Principal known constituents: essential oil = 50 to 60% anethol, fenchone, estragol, camphene, phellandrene.

Properties (analogous to those of aniseed, caraway, coriander):
1. *root:*
   - dechloridising and azoturic *diuretic* (Leclerc) for "those who can only piss a drop at a time" (Dioscorides)
   - *carminative*
   - *emmenagogue*

2. *seeds and essence:*
   - digestive stimulant
   - apéritif
   - dechloridising and azoturic diuretic
   - general tonic
   - *emmenagogue*
   - expectorant
   - antispasmodic
   - laxative
   - galactagogue
   - vermifuge
   - resolvent

Indications:
   Internal use:
1. *root*
   - *oliguria*
   - *urinary stones*
   - inflammation of the urinary tract (cystitis)
   - gout

125

2. *seeds and essence*
   - *flatulence*
   - loss of appetite
   - *dyspepsia (atonic)*, sluggish digestion
   - aerophagy, intestinal spasm
   - oliguria, urinary stones, gout
   - scanty menstrual periods
   - pulmonary diseases
   - influenza (prophylactic)
   - gastric pains, nervous vomiting
   - insufficiency of milk in nursing mothers
   - intestinal parasites

   External use:
   - congestion or engorgement of the breasts, bruises, tumours (leaves)
   - deafness
   - care of gums

Methods of use:

1. *root:*
   - decoction: 25g to 1 litre of water. Boil for 2 minutes and infuse for 10. Take 3 cups a day (oliguria, gout).
   - *syrup* of 5 roots (of butcher's broom, wild celery, parsley, fennel and asparagus): 60 to 100g per day (diuretic)

2. *seeds:*
   - powdered seeds: 1 to 4g a day
   - infusion: 1 teaspoonful per cup. Infuse for 10 minutes. One cupful after each meal
   - prophylactic against influenza: chew fennel seeds

3. *essence:*
   - essential oil: 1 to 5 drops in honey water 2 or 3 times a day
   - *carminative mixture* (to relieve flatulence):

tincture of fennel	
tincture of caraway.............................	5g of each
tincture of angelica.............................	
tincture of coriander.............................	

     50 drops in a spoonful of water or a little weak tea, after meals.
   - *a drink for urinary stones:* boil a handful of beard of maize for a few seconds in 1 litre of water. leave to infuse, adding 2 teaspoonsful of fennel seeds. Allow to cool and strain. Drink as desired.
   - *dentifrice* (strengthens the gums):

pulverised fennel seeds	
charcoal from poplar wood........................	equal parts
grey quinquina	

4. *leaves*
   - in an infusion (30g to a litre). One glass after meals (nervine and digestive tonic).
   - fresh leaves: use in resolvent poultices on bruises, tumours and congestion of the breasts.

5. *leaves, roots, seeds and essence:*
   - to treat *deafness*, direct the steam from the decoction with a funnel into the ear canal.

N.B.
1. In high doses, fennel causes convulsions (in direct contrast to aniseed). The essence makes animals timid.
2. The seeds are classed as one of the "four warming seeds" along with aniseed, caraway and coriander.
3. Fennel used to be regarded as anti-venomous (against snake-bites and scorpions), by the Chinese and Hindus; it was also held to be an excellent ophthalmic remedy and was used as a slimming agent.
4. Fennel essence is an ingredient of many liqueurs including ratafia "of the four seeds" (with angelica, celery and coriander), of compound liquorice powder, dentifrices and mouthwashes.

Garlic

Allium sativum

Liliaceae

A plant whose seasoning properties have been recognised since the most ancient times. It was Galen's "theriac of the peasant" (i.e. antidote to venomous bites, etc). In Egypt it was elevated to the status of a divinity. The workers who built the Pyramids were issued a daily clove of garlic on account of its antiseptic and tonic properties. The Hebrews, Greeks and Romans regarded garlic as a panacea.

Garlic grows wild in Spain, Sicily, Egypt and Algeria. It is cultivated in France.

Parts used: the bulb, both in cooking and in a variety of medical preparations; the *essence* is also used.

Principal known constituents: a sulphuretted glucoside, a *volatile* oil consisting of a mixture of approximately pure sulphide and oxide of allyl (Wertheim), sulphur, iodine, silica, starch, two antibiotic principles (allicine and garlicine – Binet), allistatines I and II which have a powerful effect against Staphylococcus.

Properties:
Internal use:
  – *intestinal and pulmonary antiseptic* (the essence is partially eliminated through the lung)
  – bacteriostatic and bactericide (internally and externally: Torotsev and Filatova)
  – *tonic* (comparable to quinquina)
  – *general stimulant (cardiotonic)*; stimulant of the *digestive* organs
  – circulatory stimulant
  – *hypotensive* (vasodilator of the arterioles and capillaries, according to Loeper) in cases of high blood pressure
  – slows down the pulse
  – antispasmodic, calmative
  – glandular restorative
  – *antisclerotic* (dissolves uric acid, thins the blood)
  – *diuretic*
  – anti-gout, anti-arthritic
  – apéritif
  – *stomachic* (activates the digestion of viscous foods)
  – carminative
  – *vermifuge*
  – febrifuge
  – preventive of cancer (A. Lorand)

External use:
- parasiticide
- vulnerary, healing
- analgesic
- corn cure
- resolvent
- general tonic

Indications:
Internal use:
- *prophylaxis and treatment of* infectious diseases (influenza epidemics, typhoid, diphtheria)
- diarrhoea, *dysentery* (Marcovici)
- *pulmonary complaints:* chronic bronchitis, tuberculosis, gangrene (Loeper and Lemierre), influenza, colds . . . (but see Note 1)
- *asthma and emphysema* (modifies bronchial secretion), difficulty in breathing
- whooping cough (Leclerc)
- general debility
- intestinal spasm
- sluggish digestion
- *arterial hypertension* (Pouillard)
- cardiac fatigue
- tachycardia
- vascular spasm, circulatory disorders
- varicose veins, haemorrhoids
- glandular imbalance, exophthalmic goitre
- *arteriosclerosis*, senescence
- plethora, hypercoagulability of the blood
- *rheumatism*, *gout*, arthritis
- oliguria
- oedema of the legs
- dropsy
- *urinary stones*
- gonorrhoea
- loss of appetite
- painful digestion
- flatulence
- *intestinal parasites (roundworm, threadworm, tapeworm)*
- preventive of cancer (by its antiputrid intestinal action)

External use:
- corns, warts, verrucas, callouses
- sores and wounds, infected wounds, ulcers
- scabies, tinea
- earache, rheumatic neuralgia

- deafness (rheumatic)
- wasp stings, insect bites
- cold abscesses, white tumours, cysts
- general debility

Methods of use:
Internal:
- regular use in salads and other foods (preferably *raw*).
- one or two cloves of garlic every morning (gout, general health) and regularly at meal times.
- a recommended system: at night, chop up two cloves of garlic with some heads of parsley and add a few drops of olive oil. Next morning spread on buttered toast or bread for breakfast.
- *tincture* of garlic at one-fiftieth: 10 to 15 drops, twice a day (maximum 30 drops in one day), in repeated treatments of a few days' duration with breaks.
- *alcoholic tincture made from the fresh bulb:* 20 to 30 drops twice a day (for chronic bronchitis, emphysema, whooping cough, hypertension).
- *volatile oil*: mixed with white wine (diuretic).
- *against intestinal parasites*: 3 to 4 *cloves* grated into a cup of boiling water or a cup of milk. Leave to steep overnight. Drink first thing in the morning; continue for three weeks.
- another vermifugal recipe: 25g in decoction for 20 minutes in a glass of water or milk. Two glasses a day for 3 to 4 days while the moon is waning. Repeat each month.
- *against tapeworm*: grate the cloves of a large root of garlic. Boil in milk for 20 minutes. Drink each morning until the worm is eliminated, eating no food until midday.
- juice of garlic (*vermifuge*): 20g in 200g of lukewarm milk first thing (on an empty stomach).
- *a vermifugal syrup:*

  cloves of garlic (crushed) 500g
  boiling water .... 1 litre

  Leave to infuse for 1 hour, then strain. Add 1kg sugar. 30 to 60g (2 to 3 tablespoonsful) first thing in the morning.

  *To neutralise the smell of garlic, chew 2 or 3 coffee beans, some seeds of cumin or aniseed, cardamom (Leclerc), an apple or a sprig of parsley.

External:
- garlic, crushed with fat and oil, produces the ointment known as *devil's mustard* which is a resolvent of *white swellings or tumours*.
- *to disinfect sores, wounds, ulcers*: a 10% solution of garlic juice with 1 to 2% alcohol; or compresses of vinegar of garlic: 30g grated garlic steeped for 10 days in $\frac{1}{2}$ litre vinegar.

- scabies, *tinea*: friction rubs with the mixture: 1 part of garlic and 2 of camphorated oil; or bathing with a decoction of garlic (6 cloves to 1 litre water).
- a mixture of 2 parts camphorated oil and 1 of garlic in friction rubs (rheumatism) or applied along the length of the spine for *weakness* and *general debility.*
- against *deafness* of rheumatic origin: place a swab of cotton-wool soaked in garlic in the ear each evening.
- as a *corn cure* (corns, warts, verrucas, callouses): crush a clove of garlic and apply in a fresh poultice at night, protecting the healthy skin with a plaster. This should produce results within a fortnight. Alternatively: apply a hot clove of garlic baked in the oven, renewing several times a day; or cut a sliver of garlic, apply to the corn and keep it there. Renew morning and evening.
- against *veruccas*, *warts* and little *cysts*: rub with a small piece of garlic several times a day. At the end of the treatment, follow with small clay poultices.
- *wasp stings*, insect bites, etc: withdraw sting if necessary, rub the spot with a piece of garlic.

N.B.
1. Garlic is unsuitable for persons suffering from minor skin diseases or irritation of the stomach or intestines, and for nursing mothers (it will spoil the milk and cause colic in the infant). It is contra-indicated where there are symptoms of pulmonary congestion – haemoptysis, dry or severe cough, fever (Leclerc).
2. According to an ancient custom, cloves of garlic worn in a sachet about the neck or kept against the navel are vermifugal and preventive of infectious diseases.
3. Several bulbs of garlic crushed into a *poultice* may be used as a substitute for mustard powder. This method is also used for various kinds of *rheumatism*, to produce a vesicle.
4. In certain areas (in particular the *Midi* in France) garlic is used as a suppository to strengthen children.
5. The following treatment has been recommended in cases of *typhoid fever*: wrap the patient's feet in a poultice of grated garlic to which crushed onions and nettles have been added. Wrap the poultice in a hot covering and renew every hour
6. In 1914, at the Metropolitan Hospital in New York, experiments in treatment were carried out on over a thousand cases of tuberculosis. Of the 56 different forms of treatment given, the results obtained by the use of garlic surpassed those of any other plant therapy.
7. *Tincture of garlic* (preparation):

bulb-roots of garlic............................... 50g
alcohol at 60°................................... 250g

Peel the bulbs of their outer covering, cut in pieces and steep for 10 days in alcohol, shaking frequently. Press. Filter.

Use: internally as an *antiseptic*, a *vasodilator* and *hypotensive*, and against sclerosis, rheumatism and asthma (for asthma, take several drops on a sugar lump at moments of crisis).

A useful recipe:
  Garlic Soup
  Take 1 clove of garlic per person and put in a saucepan with a little water, salt and pepper. Simmer gently. When the cloves are well cooked, crush them thoroughly. Break an egg (allowing one egg for two people) and whisk with a little water. Gradually beat in part of the garlic purée, a little at a time, then pour the mixture on to the rest of the purée in the pan, stirring well. Add sufficient warm water to make the quantity required, cover and heat gently. Put *croûtons* fried in butter into a soup tureen and strain the liquid over them. This soup is said to be a vascular tonic and a tonic for the nervous system. It is indicated in winter for respiratory illnesses (asthma, bronchitis, colds, etc. For the Provençal soup *Aïgo-bouide*, see under *Sage* (Note 4).

Some useful tips:
a) to prevent fruit from rotting: keep open containers with cloves of garlic cut in two in your fruit bowl (onion will do as well).
b) as a substitute for glue: rub the surfaces you wish to stick with a clove of garlic. Put together and hold in place.
c) to drill glass: dilute 50g oxalic acid in 25g essence of turpentine. Add 3 cloves of garlic, grated, and leave to steep for a week. Keep in a corked bottle and shake from time to time. Put a spot on the required place and drill without exerting undue pressure, adding another drop every so often as needed

Geranium

Pelargonium odorantissimum

Geraniaceae

Origin: Algeria, Réunion, Madagascar and Guinea.

There are now more than twenty genera and over 700 different species of the geranium family. Herb Robert (*Geranium robertianum*), a common British variety, has certain properties comparable to those of *P. odorantissimum*.

Parts used: the whole plant in an infusion; also the essential oil obtained by steam distillation. The Ancients regarded it as a quite exceptional vulnerary with the power to mend fractures and eliminate cancers.

Principal known constituents: resin, gallic tannin, essential oil: geraniol, citronellol, linalol, terpineol and alcohol.

Properties
Internal uses:
− tonic
− *astringent*
− haemostatic
− antiseptic (intestinal)
− *antidiabetic*
− anticancer (?)

External use:
− cicatrising
− antiseptic
− analgesic
− parasiticide
− *insect repellent (mosquitos, gnats)*

Indications:
Internal use:
− various forms of *debility* (deficiency of adrenal cortex)
− diarrhoea
− *gastro-enteritis*
− *uterine haemorrhage*, haemoptysis (decoction of leaves)
− sterility
− jaundice
− *diabetes*
− *urinary stones*
− *gastric ulcer*
− cancer (?)

External use:
− engorgement or congestion of the breasts
− sores, burns
− *cancerous conditions*, cancer of the uterus (?)

- *tonsillitis*, inflammations of mouth, *throat* and tongue (stomatitis, glossitis, thrush, etc)
- ophthalmia
- facial neuralgia
- gastric and lumbar pain
- oedema of the legs
- dermatosis (herpes, dry eczema); shingles, scurf
- lice
- insect repellent (mosquitos, gnats, etc)

Methods of use:
Internal:
- *infusion:* 1 dessertspoonful to 1 cup of boiling water. Infuse for 10 minutes. Drink 3 cups a day between meals.
- *essential oil:* 2 to 4 drops 2 or 3 times a day in honey water or in alcoholic solution

External:
- a handful to 1 litre of water. Boil for 10 minutes. Use as a *gargle* to treat tonsillitis, inflammations of mouth, throat and tongue.
  In conjunction with this treatment, paint on this medication:

  liquid extract of Herb Robert 5g
  rose honey 60g
  distilled water 25g
  (Leclerc)
- bruised leaves, applied to cuts and sores, aid the healing process.
- crushed fresh flowers – or leaves – in applications for ophthalmia.
- decoction, or applications of the cooked plant, for facial neuralgia, gastric and lumbar pain, oedema of the legs, congested breasts, herpes, dry eczema.
- the essence in association with other essences in the treatment of burns, sores, shingles and as a gargle for sore throat, tonsillitis.
- see under *Origanum* for a formula for an ointment to treat lice.

N.B.
Italy – Discovery of an anticoagulant principle in the leaves of several species of geranium.
Dr. Simone Vetrano of the Sciacca Institute of Marine Biology has detected the presence of an anticoagulant principle in the leaves of many species of the genus *Pelargonium*, in particular those of certain ornamental varieties of geranium. This substance has, *in vitro*, a persistent anticoagulant affect on human blood. Experiments on animals have resulted in no cases of haemorrhage, no signs of toxicity nor parenchymatous alterations. (*Présse Medicale* 1962).

Ginger

Zingiber officinale

Zingiberaceae

Native of India, China and Java. Grown in the Philippines and Tahiti.
   One of the most highly esteemed spices and drugs from ancient times to the Middle Ages.

Parts used:
root, essence obtained from the roots by steam distillation.

Principal known constituents:
an oleo-resin containing gingenol, composed of several phenols, ginger-one and zingiberene.

Properties:
   Internal use:
   – apértif
   – stomachic
   – carminative
   – antiseptic
   – stimulant
   – tonic
   – antiscorbutic
   – febrifuge

   External use:
   – *analgesic*
   – *ophthalmic (?)*

Indications:
   Internal use:
   – loss of appetite
   – painful digestion, dyspepsia
   – flatulence
   – diarrhoea
   – prevention of contagious diseases
   – impotence
   – scurvy

   External use:
   – rheumatic pains
   – sore throat, tonsillitis, angina
   – cataract (see Note 2)
   – contusions (see Note 5)

Methods of use:
Internal:
- seasoning, used in cooking and pastry-making (in England, Germany and many Eastern countries).
- *essence*: 1 to 3 drops several times a day in honey water.
- *tincture*: 10 to 20 drops before meals, taken either alone or in combination as follows:

tincture of ginger................................	10g
tincture of wormwood	5g
	(Leclerc)

20 to 30 drops before meals.

External:
- *rheumatic pains*: friction rubs with liniment:

tincture of ginger................................	40g
essence of origanum	2g
spirit of rosemary	60
	(Leclerc)

My own formula:

tincture of ginger................................	180g
essence of origanum	6g
essence of juniper	6g
essence of cypress	3g
essence of turpentine	12g
spirit of rosemary	500ml

Use in friction rubs 2 or 3 times a day on the painful areas. Continue for 2 to 3 weeks, even if the pain has disappeared after 2 or 3 days.

- inflammation of the throat, with accompanying oedema: gargles with $\frac{1}{2}$ to 1 teaspoon of tincture of ginger to 1 cup of lukewarm boiled water.

N.B.
1. Ginger is used in the making of many drinks: ginger beer, ginger brandy, Jamaica ginger, etc.
2. Distilled ginger water has in the past been regarded as one of the best ophthalmic remedies (cataract).
3. Women in Senegal and Fouta-Djalon use the tubers of the ginger plant in the making of belts with the aim of arousing the dormant senses of their husbands (G. Capus and D. Bois).
4. Ginger is also used in powdered form "in local rectal applications to persuade horses to keep their tails raised, a sign of strength and good breeding appreciated by the discerning members of the equestrian fraternity" (Leclerc).
5. See under *Cinnamon* for aromatic tincture of arnica (contusions).

Hyssop

Hyssopus officinalis

Labiatae

An indigenous plant, common in the Midi region of France and cultivated in gardens as an aromatic and medicinal herb. The Hebrews called
it *Ezob*, from which the name hyssop is derived, holding it sacred.
Hippocrates used it in treating pleurisy, Dioscorides for dyspnoea and
asthma (in hyssop wine, or 'cooked in water' as a decoction).

It may be used in the form of infusions (of the leaves and flowering
tops) or the essential oil obtained by distillation of the plant.

Principal known constituents:

hyssopine, saponine, choline (2g %), silica, potassium nitrate, tannin,
essential oil: phellandrene, borneol, pino-camphone, thujone, limonene
and geraniol.

Because it contains ketones (pino-camphone), though in infinitesimal
quantities, the essence is toxic in high doses, causing *epileptic attacks* in
those so predisposed (Cadéac and Meunier; in Caujolle's opinion it is the
only herbal essence capable of producing a true epileptic attack in man).
Nevertheless its toxicity is far less than that of wormwood.

Properties:

Internal use:
- *eases and modifies expectoration.* Counteracts stasis of bronchial
  secretions (the essence is eliminated via the lungs)
- antiseptic, bactericide
- *antitussive*, emollient
- stimulation (*of the medulla oblongata*: Cadéac and Meunier)
- hypertensive (Caujolle, Cazal)
- sudorific, diuretic
- digestive, stomachic
- emmenagogue
- *vermifuge*
- anticancer (?)

External use:
- cicatrising, resolvent

Indications:

Internal use:
- *asthma*, hay fever, dyspnoea (difficulty in breathing)
- *chronic bronchitis*, cough, influenza

- tuberculosis (the essence neutralises the tuberculosis bacillus in a dose of 0.2 parts per thousand)
- loss of appetite
- dermatosis
- rheumatism
- hypotension (low blood pressure)
- *urinary stones*
- eruptive fevers
- dyspepsia, sluggish digestion
- gastralgia, colic, distension of the stomach
- scanty periods
- leucorrhoea
- intestinal parasites
- malignant conditions (?)

External use:
- wounds, bruises
- syphilides, cancerous growths, eczema

Methods of use:
Internal:
- *infusion*: 20g to 1 litre water. Three cupfuls a day. In the treatment of bronchitis it can be used in conjunction with the flowers of marsh mallow, blue mallow and mullein.
- *alcoholic tincture*: 10 to 30 drops in half a glass of water.
- *anti-asthmatic herbal tea:*

root of wild celery.................................	⎫
root of burdock.....................................	⎬ 30g of each
root of couch-grass.................................	⎭
root of elecampane.................................	
leaves of maidenhair fern 30g	
horehound...	⎫ 3g of each
hyssop	⎭
fennel (seeds)......................................	15g

Boil for 3 minutes in a litre of water. Take as a normal drink.

- *essential oil*: 2 to 4 drops in honey water in alcoholic suspension 3 times a day

External:
- *infusion*: 30g per litre of water. Used in washes and compresses (wounds). Hyssop is one of the ingredients of *The herbal elixir of Grand-Chartreuse:*

```
fresh lemon balm ................................. 640g
fresh hyssop....................................... 640g
fresh angelica..................................... 320g
cinnamon........................................... 160g
saffron ............................................ 40g
mace............................................... 40g
```

Steep for 8 days in 10 litres of alcohol, press and distill over a quantity of fresh plants – lemon balm and hyssop. After a certain time add 1,250g of sugar and filter

Another formula:

```
essence of lemon balm.............................. 2g
essence of hyssop ................................. 2g
essence of angelica ............................... 10g
essence of peppermint ............................. 20g
essence of nutmeg.................................. 2g
essence of clove................................... 2g
alcohol at 80°..................................... 2 litres
sugar.............................................. to taste
```

It is coloured either yellow, with a few drops of tincture of saffron, or green, with a few drops of dissolved indigo or alcohol tincture of elder leaves.

Juniper

Juniperus communis

Coniferae

A small hardwood bush found in Central and Southern Europe, Sweden and Canada, etc. Known since antiquity for its antiseptic and diuretic properties (Cato the Elder).

Parts used:
berries, wood, leaves and essence obtained by steam distillation of the berries.

Principal known constituents:
juniperine; an essential oil containing borneol and isoborneol, cadinene, pinene, camphene, terpineol, terpenic alcohol – juniper camphor, albumin, sugar (73%).

Properties:
Internal use:
- *tonic* (of visceral functions, of the *nervous system*, of the *digestive tract*); *general stimulant of secretions* (berries), apéritif
- *antiseptic* (pulmonary, intestinal, urinary, haemal – i.e. of the blood)
- *stomachic*
- *depurative* (purifying)
- *diuretic* (uricolytic – sudorific): the wood
- antirheumatic: promotes excretion of *uric acid* and toxins, *antigout*
- *antidiabetic*
- emmenagogue
- soporific

External use:
- parasiticide
- depurative (purifying)
- antiseptic
- cicatrising

Indications:
Internal use:
- general or organal *lassitude* (sluggish digestion)
- loss of appetite
- prophylactic of contagious diseases
- diseases of the *urinary tract* (kidneys, bladder): *gonorrhoea*, cystitis, (do not use in cases of acute inflammation of the kidneys)

- albuminuria
- oliguria
- dropsy, cirrhosis
- intestinal fermentations
- *urinary stones*
- arteriosclerosis
- *gout*
- *rheumatism*, arthritis
- *diabetes*
- *painful menstruation*, leucorrhoea

External use:
- after-effects of *paralysis*
- weeping eczema, acne
- sores, atonic wounds, ulcers
- dermatosis, toothache (Cade oil)
- canine mange (veterinary use)
- domestic disinfectant

Methods of use:
Internal:
- *berries:* 1. infusion: 20 to 30g per litre of water, or 1 teaspoonful to a cup. Infuse for 10 minutes. 3 cups a day (*diuretic* and *stomachic*).
  Among the ingredients of the wines *Trousseau* and *Charité*.
  2. The berries have *antidiabetic* properties when taken as follows: grind about 10 berries and take them with water daily for from 2 weeks to a month. Repeat at further intervals.
- "mother-tincture" of berries: 15 drops in an infusion, after meals.
- *aqueous extract*: 1 to 5g a day in either a draught or pills.
- *essence*: from 2 to 5 drops per day in alcholic solution, or in honey water.
- *syrup to treat arthritis:*

  soft extract of juniper berries 10g
  liquid extract of horsetail.......................... 10g
  syrup of 5 roots (see under *Fennel*) 400g
  2 to 5 tablespoonsful a day.

- *juniper wine:*

  crushed berries 30g
  chopped stalks.................................. 15g
  white wine..................................... 1 litre
  Leave to steep for 4 days. Strain and add 30g sugar.
  Take between a liqueur glass and a tumberful a day (*tonic, apéritif,*

diuretic, anticalculous (anti-urinary stones) and indicated for *autumn fevers*). The tonic effect is strengthened with the addition of a pinch of lesser wormwood and 15g of wild horseradish root.

– another formula for juniper wine:

crushed berries	75g
white mustard seed	7.5g
white wine	1 litre

Leave to steep for 5 days. Filter. Take ½ a glass twice daily (tonic, apéritif, stomachic).

– diuretic wine from the Hôtel-Dieu, or Trousseau:

digitalis	5g
scilla	15g
juniper berries	25g
potassium acetate	50g
alcohol	100g
white wine	900g

(20g contains 0.10g of digitalis)

External:
– juniper wood: 50g per litre of water in decoction. Use to bathe *torpid wounds* and *lingering ulcers* – promotes healing.
– stimulant liniment for *paralysis:*

essence of juniper	2g
menthol	1g
essence of turpentine	20g
90° alcohol	120g

– juniper baths (rheumatism, arthritis): sometimes bring about spectacular results. Also used for washing.
– see under *Rosemary* for a formula for an aphrodisiac bath.
– the grilled *berries* make an excellent *domestic disinfectant.*
– see under *Ginger* for a formula for friction rubs.

N.B.
1. Juniper essence readily dissolves iodine which then loses its normal reactions (it no longer colours starch blue nor the skin yellow). When the essence of iodised juniper is absorbed, the iodine is rapidly released to reappear in the urine and nasal mucus (Heller). This gives additional proof of the rapid dispersal of essences throughout the organism.
2. It is strongly recommended that the berries used in cooking (sauerkraut) should themselves be eaten. Only the snobbish leave them on the side of the plate.

3. Distillation yields spirits of juniper.
4. Young shoots, dried on a wicker screen, chopped into small pieces and kept in an airtight container, provide an excellent tea.
5. *Cade oil* is extracted from the trunk of mature juniper trees. It is used in the treatment of dermatosis and toothache (a little piece of cotton-wool soaked in the oil is placed on the offending tooth).
6. Oil of Haarlem is also extracted from juniper, but its other ingredients remain a secret (bay berries and pine wood?).
7. Juniper essence imparts a scent of violets to urine.

Lavender

Lavendula officinalis

Labiatae

A very valuable plant, common in the Midi region of France, in Italy and Dalmatia where it is found at an altitude of between 700 and 1,400 metres (2,000 to 4,000 feet), French lavender – the oldest known variety – being the most highly valued. Lavender is endowed with many felicitous properties.

Parts used:
flowers and essential oil obtained by steam distillation of the plant (in France, the annual production of lavender essence yields between 75,000 and 150,000kg).

Principal known constituents:
essence – ethers of linalyl and geranyl (35 to 55% of linalyl acetate), geraniol, linalol, cineol, d-borneol, limonene, l-pinene, caryophyllene, butyric and valeric esters, coumarin.

Properties:
Internal use:
- *antispasmodic* (it is excitant at toxic doses)
- analgesic, *calmative of cerebro-spinal excitability* (taken both internally and cutaneously): Cadéac and Meunier
- internal and external antiseptic, *bactericide* (J. Marchand, Forgues and P. Neurisse)
- pulmonary *antiseptic*: modifies bronchial secretions, antitussive
- cholagogue, choleretic (Chabrol)
- *diuretic*, sudorific
- tonic, restorative, cardiotonic and calmative for the nerves of the heart
- antirheumatic
- increases gastric secretion, intestinal stimulant
- *antimigraine*
- *vermifuge*
- emmenagogue
- hypotensive (Caujolle, Cazal)

External use:
- cicatrising
- antiseptic, disinfectant

144

- *parasiticide, insecticide*
- antivenomous
- regulator of nervous system

Indications:

Internal use:
- irritability, spasm, insomnia
- eruptive fevers, *infectious diseases*
- melancholia, general physical and mental debility, anxiety
- *respiratory ailments: asthma, spasmodic cough* (whooping-cough), influenza, bronchitis, tuberculosis, pneumonia
- *oliguria*
- rheumatism
- infantile debility
- gastric atony (sluggish digestion), intestinal atony (flatulence)
- *migraine*, *vertigo*, hysteria, *after-effects of paralysis*, nervous crises
- *enteritis*, diarrhoea, typhoid, *intestinal spasm*
- cystitis, *gonorrhoea*
- scrofulosis, chlorosis
- intestinal parasites
- scanty menstrual periods
- *leucorrhoea*
- hypertension (high blood pressure)

External use:
- *wounds and sores* of all descriptions: simple, atonic (leg ulcers), infected, gangrenous, syphylitic; chancres, anal fistula
- chronic perineal and peri-anal eczema
- leucorrhoea
- *burns*
- pulmonary diseases; sinusitis, influenza, bronchitis (see under *Eucalyptus*)
- acne, acne rosacea
- *insect bites*, animal and adder bites (first-aid)
- lice, scabies
- alopecia

Methods of use:

Internal:
- *infusion:* 1 dessertspoonful of flowers to 1 cup boiling water. Infuse for 10 minutes. 3 cups a day between meals.
- *alcoholic tincture:* 40 drops, 4 times a day, in a little water (diuretic)
- *essential oil:* 2 to 5 drops in honey water or in alcoholic solution 2 to 3 times a day. As an analgesic, 1g taken on an empty stomach reduces sensitivity, leaving the mind alert but relaxed.

145

- *treatment of venereal disease:* capsules or *perles* of deterpenated lavender at a strength of 0.05 to 0.10cg for 2 to 10 days in the treatment of *gonorrhoea* (antiseptic/analgesic, preferable to the essences of sandalwood, cedar or copaiba).
- *infusion of 5 flowers:* diuretic in *infectious diseases*, eruptive fevers (Leclerc):

lavender flowers	10g
marigold flowers	5g
borage flowers	5g
broom flowers	5g
wild pansy flowers	5g

1 tablespoonful to a glass of boiling water. Infuse for 10 minutes. 3 glasses a day.

External:
- *decoction:* a handful of flowers to a litre of water. Boil for 10 minutes. Add a further litre of water (used in vaginal douches for *leucorrhoea*).
- a handful of flowers in ½ a litre olive oil. Place over a bain-marie for 2 hours. Leave to steep overnight. Strain through muslin. Anoint in the treatment of dry ezcema.
- *spirit:* in lotions and friction rubs for rheumatism.
- *essence:* for washing, irrigating and dressing *wounds*, *sores* and *burns*:

essence of deterpenated lavender	100g
sulphoricinate of soda (33%)	900g

to be used at a dose of 2 to 4% in water. Equally as a disinfectant spray in *public places* (2% solution).
- bactericidal combinations (*atonic wounds*)

{ essence of thyme
{ essence of lavender

or

{ essence of lavender
{ essence of deterpenated lemon
{ carvacrol

- equally, for wounds and burns: the essence of lavender is combined with other essences in the product *Solvarome*, used in straightforward application or diluted in water.
- aromatic oil to be painted on to *atonic wounds*:

essence of lavender	10g
olive oil	100g

- *syphilitic sores, chancres, anal fistulae, alopeeia:* light application of deterpenated essence.
- *vaginal discharge (leucorrhoea), feminine hygiene:*

```
        powdered borax ..............................  100g
        essence of deterpenated lavender...................  5g
```
Divide into 10g sachets. Dissolve 1 sachet in a litre of warm water for a vaginal douche.

– *Helmerich's ointment* (against *scabies):*
```
        gum tragacanth...................................  1g
        sub-carbonate of potassium ......................  50g
        sublimate sulphur...............................  100g
        glycerine.......................................  200g
        essence of lavender.............................
        essence of lemon................................
        essence of peppermint ..........................  } 1g of each
        essence of clove................................
        essence of cinnamon ............................
```

– *ointment for anal fissures (Meurisse):*
```
        deterpenated lavender ...........................  1g
        liquid paraffin..................................  5g
        zinc oxide.......................................  10g
        subnitrate of bismuth............................  4g
        white vaseline ..................................  15g
```

– *Sabouraud's stimulating lotion:*
```
        tincture of essence of lavender .....................  30g
        pure acetone ....................................  30g
        distilled water ..................................  30g
        pure sodium nitrate ............................0.50g
        pilocarpine nitrate .............................  50g
        alcohol at 90°...................................  250cc
```
Use daily as a scalp rub.

– *insect bites:* rub the bite with a mixture of equal parts of the essence of lavender and alcohol.
– *decoction* or 'milk' of lavender for *general baths* (for weak and delicate children). These baths are *sedative* (nervous troubles, insomnia). Take preferably at night and alternate with baths of rosemary, pine, calamus and seaweed.

Aspic, or Spike Lavender (*Lavandula spica*), is a variety that grows by the seaside and to an altitude of 500–600 metres, yielding *spike oil* (used as a cerebro-spinal tranquilliser).

Spike oil, unlike essence of *lavandula officinalis*, contains few esters (lynalyl acetate). But it does contain a more or less important quantity of camphor. It is used chiefly as an insecticide and in the varnishing industry.

147

Insects have, in addition, created the hybrid *Lavandin*.

A particularly fine species of lavender is found in the area of Mitcham in Surrey.

N.B.

1. The essence of lavender has antivenous properties well-known to hunters in certain regions. In the Alps, if their dogs are bitten by adders, huntsmen will get lavender, crush it and rub it on the bites. The venom is neutralised immediately.

2. At a strength of 4.5% the essence of lavender kills Eberth's bacillus (typhoid) and staphylococcus. At 5% it will destroy Loeffler's bacillus (diphtheria) (Professors Morel and Rochaix, 1926). Its antiseptic power is greater than those of phenol, cresol and guiaicol.

3. Lavender essence kills the tuberculosis bacillus at a stength of 0.2% (Professors Courmont, Morel and Bay, 1928). Lavender vapour destroys pnuemococcus and haemolytic streptococcus in 12 to 24 hours.

4. In antiquity, lavender water was used to combat *blepharitis* (inflammation of the eyelids).

5. Lavender water:
   fresh lavender flowers 60g
   32° alcohol.................................... 1 litre

   Leave to macerate for a month, then filter.

6. Lavender flowers are used to keep linen fragrant and keep away the moths.

7. See under *Eucalyptus* for the formula for inhalations; under *Clove* for the formula for English aromatic vinegar.

8. Lavender is widely used in certain proprietary bath preparations.

Lavender-cotton

Santolina chamaecyparissus

Compositae

Sometimes confusingly, called French lavender. Grows in the mountain regions of Europe, and has been introduced into domestic gardens.

Parts used:
seeds, essential oil.

Properties:
- *vermifuge* (analogous to tansy and *semen-contra*, i.e. capitules of Artemisia, e.g. santonica): Galen, Murray
- stimulant
- antispasmodic
- emmenagogue

Indications:
- Ascaris (roundworm)
- Oxyuris (pinworm, threadworm)

Methods of use:
- *seeds*: 1 dessertspoonful to a cup of boiling water. Infuse for 10 minutes. 1 cup every morning for a week while the moon is waning. Repeat for 3 months.
- *powdered seeds*: tablets of 0.50g (between 4 and 8 a day), or 2 to 4g in honey.
- *essential oil*: 3 to 10 drops in capsules 2 or 3 times a day, or take on a sugar-lump. Drink plenty afterwards.
- *vermifuge for children* (Leclerc):
  powdered seeds of lavender-cotton 2g
  syrup of peach flowers 30g
  honey preparation 70g

Lemon

Citrus limonum

Rutaceae

Thought to have its origin in India. Grows in Southern Europe, especially in Spain and Portugal.

The fruit is used in various kinds of preparation, or the essence itself, obtained by expression of the outer part of the fresh rind (the lemon contains numerous large pockets of essence in the subepidermic parenchyma). Green fruit yields more essence than ripe fruit. About 3,000 lemons are needed to produce 1 kilo of essence. The pulp is used to prepare citric acid.

Principal known constituents:
- 30% juice which itself contains between 6 and 8% citric acid, malic acid, citrates of lime and potassium
- *glucides*: glucose and fructose (directly assimilable), sucrose
- mineral salts and trace elements: calcium, iron, silica, phosphorus, manganese and copper
- gums – mucilage – albumins
- vitamins, especially B (B_1, B_2, B_3); also vitamins A, C and PP.

  Vitamins B_1, B_2 and B_3 play an important part in nutrition and in maintaining the balance of the nervous system.

  Carotene (provitamin A) is found chiefly in the skin, vitamin A in the fresh pulp and juice. These are extremely important in the process of growing and in maintaining tissue vitality.

  Vitamin C (40 to 50mg per 100g of fruit) plays a vital role in the processes of oxygen reduction and influences the endocrine glands.

  Vitamin PP is a factor in the protection of the vascular system.
- the *essence* contains approximately 95% terpenes (pinene, limonene, phellandrene, camphene, sesquiterpenes), linalol, acetates of linalyl and geranyl, citral and citronellal (6 to 8%), aldehydes and a camphor of lemon.

Properties:
These are numerous. In Spain and certain other countries the lemon is used in the treatment of countless conditions, systematically and with obvious success.

Internal use:
- *bactericide* (see Note 1), *antiseptic*
- activates the white corpuscles in the defence of the organism
- cooling, refreshing

- febrifuge
- tonic for the nervous and sympathetic nervous system
- cardiotonic
- alkalising agent (Rancoule – see Note 8)
- diuretic
- *antirheumatic, antigout* (Labbé), anti-arthritic
- calmative, combats excess gastric acidity (see Note 8), anti-spasmodic
- *antisclerotic* (combats the ageing process)
- *antiscorbutic*
- *venous tonic*
- lowers hyperviscosity of the blood
- hypotensive
- depurative
- rectifies mineral deficiencies
- antianaemic (haemopoietic)
- aids *gastro-hepatic* and pancreatic secretions (hepatic and pancreatic stimulant)
- haemostatic
- carminative
- vermifuge
- *antidotal*
- antipruriginous
- the *rind* is tonic and carminative
- the seeds are antihelminthic (vermifuge) and febrifuge

External use:
- *antiseptic*, antitoxic
- antipruriginous
- cicatrising
- astringent
- antidotal (insect bites), parasiticide
- care of the skin
- insect repellent (clothes moths, ants)

Indications:
  Internal use:
- *infections* of many kinds (pulmonary, intestinal, etc)
- infectious diseases (stimulates "curative leucocytosis")
- malaria, feverish states (Cazin)
- the prevention of epidemics
- debility, loss of appetite
- ascites (Binet and Tanret)
- *rheumatism*, arthritis, gout
- urinary and gallstones
- gastric hyperacidity, stomach ulcers, gastritis
- dyspepsia (painful digestion), aerophagy

151

- *scurvy*
- *arteriosclerosis*
- *varicose veins*, phlebitis, capillary fragility
- *plethora, hyperviscosity of the blood* (lemon treatment "does as well as bleeding")
- obesity
- hypertension (high blood pressure)
- pulmonary tuberculosis, tuberculosis of the spine (Pott's disease)
- demineralisation, growing pains, convalescence
- anaemia
- *jaundice, vomiting* (Avicenne)
- hepatic and pancreatic deficiency
- hepatic congestion
- haemophilia
- haemorrhage (nosebleed, gastric and intestinal haemorrhage, haemoptysis, haematuria)
- meteorism, flatulence
- dystentery, diarrhoea, typhoid
- intestinal parasites (Oxyuris)
- also: asthma, bronchitis, influenza, pneumonia, gonorrhoea, syphilis, senescence, headache

External use:
- head colds, sinusitis, sore throat, tonsillitis, otitis (inflammation of the ear), gingivitis
- nosebleed
- inflammations of mouth and tongue (stomatitis, thrush, glossitis): Leven
- buccal syphilides (Caussade and Goubeau)
- blepharitis (inflammation of the eyelids)
- eruptions, boils, minor skin conditions
- migraine
- verrucas, warts
- herpes (Berlureaux)
- chilblains
- infected and putrid wounds
- insect bites
- snake bites (first-aid)
- tinea, scabies
- skin and beauty care
- facial seborrhoea, freckles
- prevention of wrinkles, hand care
- brittle nails
- tender feet
- to repel ants and clothes moths
- to purify drinking water

Methods of use:

Internal:

- lemonade (slices of fresh lemon in water, or the juice of a lemon in half a glass of sugared water); lemonade is recommended for patients with fever and in cases of vomiting or haemorrhaging.
- lemon juice: the treatment should be carried out by increasing the dose progressively from ½ a lemon to 10 or 12 lemons daily and then decreasing at the same rate over a period of 4 to 5 weeks; thereafter 1 or 2 lemons daily (use very ripe fruit).
- *vermifuge:* crush the rind, pulp and seeds of 1 lemon. Leave to steep for 2 hours in water with honey added. Express. Drink at bedtime.
- a *decoction* of the whole fruit is also indicated in the treatment of *worms.*
- against *Oxyuris* (threadworm): the pips ground up and taken with honey first thing each morning.
- for *congestion of the liver:* pour boiling water over 3 chopped lemons at night and drink first thing the next morning.
- to counteract putting on weight: pour one cup of boiling water on to 2 heads of camomile and one lemon (sliced) and leave to macerate overnight. Strain and drink first thing in the morning.
- an infusion is also indicated for *aerophagy.*
- *essence:* 5 to 10 drops in honey water or in a draught.

External:

- for *head colds, sinusitis:* a few drops of juice in the nostrils, several times a day.
- for *nosebleeds:* a pad of cotton-wool soaked in lemon juice.
- for *thrush, stomatitis:* lemon, honey and water, in prolonged mouthwashes.
- for sore throat, *tonsillitis:* gargle with the juice of a lemon in a glass of warm water.
- in *the eyes of newborn babies* and against *blepharitis:* 1 or 2 drops of lemon juice.
- on the forehead, for *migraine:* compresses of lemon juice; or slices of lemon on the temples.
- on *cuts* and *infected wounds* (antiseptic, haemostatic): lemon juice either neat or diluted.
- against *chilblains:* rub with lemon juice (also as a preventive).
- for *otitis:* lemon juice in the ears.
- for *warts and verrucas:* paint twice a day with strong vinegar in which the rinds of two lemons have been macerated for 8 days.
- for *brittle nails:* apply lemon juice, morning and night, for a week.
- for *greasy skin:* soak a piece of cotton-wool in lemon juice and bathe the face morning and night (allow to dry for 20 minutes before applying cream or powder).

- against *freckles*: slightly salted lemon juice as a face lotion.
- to banish *wrinkles*: apply lemon juice as a face lotion twice a week, rubbing in well (also clears the skin).
- to *keep the hands soft*: rub with a mixture of:

  lemon juice ....
  glycerine. .... } equal parts
  eau de Cologne ....

- to *keep teeth white*: brush once a week with lemon juice.
- for *tender feet*: bathe in lime-blossom water, then rub with lemon juice.
- for *insect bites* rub with a slice of lemon. May also be used on snake-bites (first-aid).

N.B.

1. The work of Morel and Rochaix on the *bactericidal action of essence of lemon* has demonstrated that:
   a) vaporised lemon essence neutralises meningococcus in 15 minutes, Eberth's bacillus (typhoid) in less than one hour, pneumococcus in between 1 and 3 hours, *Staphylococcus aureus* in 2 hours and haemolytic streptococcus in from 3 to 12 hours.
   b) the essence neutralises Eberth's bacillus in 5 minutes, staphylococcus in 5 minutes, Loeffler's bacillus (diphtheria)'in 20 minutes, and renders tuberculosis bacillus completely inactive at a strength of 0.2%.

   A few drops will kill 92% of all bacteria in oysters within 15 minutes: Charles Richet.

2. Lemon juice may be used to disinfect doubtful drinking water (the juice of one lemon to a litre) and meat or fish of dubious freshness.
3. To make *curdled milk* with lemon juice: add the juice of a lemon, drop by drop, to a pint (or half a litre) of milk, stirring continuously. The process is completed when the milk adopts a granular texture. The resulting substance is very rich in vitamins.
4. To make *lemonade*: slice one lemon and put in a cask with 5 litres of water. Shake twice a day. After 8 days, strain and bottle. Seal the bottles and store on their sides.
5. An infusion of the peel of 2 or 3 lemons to a litre of water makes an excellent drink *for immediate consumption*. Add a few drops of fresh lemon juice.
6. *A lemonade purgative*:

   magnesium carbonate 11g
   citric acid. 18g
   water. 300g

   Flavour with tincture of lemon.
7. Lemon is an ingredient of compound spirits of lemon balm.
8. *The acidity of lemon*: it may come as a surprise to read that lemon is both an alkalising agent and a gastric antacid. Rancoule and Labbé have dealt with this aspect at length. The acid taste does not in fact

signify that lemon has an acidic effect on the organism, since it is due to organic acids which do not remain acidic at cellular level. Experiments have proved that prolonged use of lemon brings about within the organism the production of potassium carbonate which neutralises excess acidity in the bodily fluids. Gastric hyperacidity may equally be normalised with lemon juice diluted with water (the lemon is in any case classed among foodstuffs basic to the diet).

Natural citric acid is oxidised during digestion. The remaining salts yield carbonates and bicarbonates of calcium and potassium which maintain the alkalinity of the blood.

Thus a substance may produce an exterior acidic reaction and yet generate alkalinity in the organism.

9. Lemons will give a greater quantity of juice if they are soaked in warm water for 5 minutes before squeezing.

Some useful hints:

- To clean tarnished brasswork, rub with ½ a lemon which has itself been rubbed with rock salt
- To clean silver jewellery, rub with a slice of lemon, rinse in warm water and dry with a chamois leather.
- To clean a white marble fireplace, rub with ½ a lemon, giving extra attention to stained areas, then rub over with a slightly oiled linen cloth.
- To remove rust spots from white linen, put a slice of lemon between 2 sheets of tissue paper, then place this on the stain and press with a hot iron. Repeat if necessary.
- To clean a stained wash-basin, rub with a mixture of ½ a cup of lemon juice and a large pinch of salt
- Fingers stained with ink, or fruit or vegetable juice, may be cleaned with lemon juice.
- To repel *clothes moths*, hang bags containing dried lemon rind in the wardrobe.
- To repel *ants*, put down a rotten lemon.

Lemongrass

Adropogon or *Cymbopogon citratus*

Gramineae

A fragrant perennial grass, it comes from India, Madagascar, Tonkin, the Antilles. Not to be confused with Lemon Verbena Oil (Lippia citriodorm).

Principal known constituents:
essence obtained by distillation, chiefly containing citral.

Properties:
Internal use:
- stomachic, gastric stimulant
- antiseptic
- regulator of the parasympathetic system
- galactagogue

External use:
- parasiticide

Indications
Internal use:
- gastric atony (sluggish digestion)
- enteritis, *colitis*
- *dystonia of the autonomic nervous system*
- insufficiency of milk

External use:
- lice

Methods of use:
Internal:
- essence: 5 drops on a sugar-lump or in alcoholic solution 2 or 3 times a day.

External:
- see under *Origanum* for the formula for an ointment to treat lice.

Marjoram

Origanum marjorana

Labiatea

Also known as sweet marjoram, knotted marjoram, pot marjoram. Indigenous to Persia, the Mediterranean coastal regions, Hungary and Yugoslavia.

Parts used:
the flowering heads, essence.

Principal known constituents:
essential oil, obtained by steam distillation: 85% mixture of camphor and borneol (Bruylants), terpinene, sabinene.

Properties:
Internal use:
– *antispasmodic,* calmative
– vagotonic (increases the tone of the parasympathetic nerves, reduces that of the sympathetic nerves); hypotensive (Caujolle)
– arterial vasodilator
– sedative, dulls the senses, causes drowsiness (in large doses the essence is stupefacient: Cadéac and Meunier)
– carminative (augments intestinal peristalsis)
– expectorant
– digestive stimulant
– anaphrodisiac

External use:
– vulnerary
– tonic (baths)
– analgesic

Indications (comparable to those of peppermint and thyme):
Internal use:
– anxiety
– *digestive spasms (aerophagy), respiratory spasms* (Leclerc)
– arteritic syndromes
– *insomnia, migraine,* tics
– *general physical and nervous debility, mental instability*
– flatulence
– genital erethism

157

External use:
- weakness, debility (baths)
- rheumatic neuralgia
- coryza (colds in the head)

Methods of use:
Internal:
- *infusion*: 1 dessertspoonful of the chopped plant to one cup of boiling water. Infuse for 10 minutes. 2 to 3 cups per day.
- *essence*: 3 or 4 drops 2 or 3 times a day, in honey water.
- *aromatic water*: 5 to 20g a day either on its own or combined with other antispasmodics:

aromatic water of marjoram	50g
aromatic water of valerian	25g
aromatic water of lettuce	25g

1 to 3 tablespoonsful at bedtime (anxiety, insomnia).

- *antispasmodic oleosaccharum:*

essence of marjoram	50 drops
white sugar	25g
lactose	25g

1 teaspoon in an infusion, at bedtime.

tincture of arnica	300 drops
spirit of mandrake root	100 drops
aromatic water of marjoram	100ml

1 teaspoon twice a day (arteritic syndromes).

External:
- marjoram is superior to thyme in *fortifying baths.*
- for colds in the head: inhale the infusion.
- for rheumatic pains: compresses soaked in the infusion; or rub with an ointment containing the essence (at a strength of 1–2%).

N.B.
1. Marjoram essence neutralises the tuberculosis bacillus at a dose of 0.4%.
2. To preserve their voices, singers throughout the ages have used a great variety of concoctions: infusions of horehound sweetened with honey, cabbage or garlic water, pellets made up of mustard powder and honey etc. An infusion of marjoram sweetened with honey is a stock remedy.

Niaouli

Melaleuca viridiflora

Myrtaceae

This tree is found in abundance in New Caledonia.

Essence of niaouli, or "gomenol", is obtained by steam distillation of the fresh leaves. For therapeutic purposes, the *purified* essence of niaouli is used.

Distillation of the leaves of various other species of *Melaleuca* yields a similar product known as *cajuput oil* (see under *Cajuput*).

Principal known constituents:
35 to 66% eucalyptol, 15% terpinol, d-pinene, l-limonene, citrene, terebenthene, valeric, acetic and butyric esters.

Properties:
Internal use:
- *antiseptic* (general, bronchial, intestinal, urinary)
- *balsamic*
- anticatarrhal
- analgesic
- vermifuge

External use:
- *tissue stimulant* (antiseptic and cicatrising)
- antiseptic

Indications:
Internal use:
- *chronic bronchitis, pulmonary tuberculosis*
- influenza, pneumonia
- *whooping cough*, asthma
- *rhinitis*, sinusitis, inflammation of the ear, nasal catarrh
- tuberculosis of the bones
- intestinal infections (enteritis, dysentery)
- urinary infections (cystitis, urethritis)
- puerperal infections
- rheumatism
- intestinal parasites

External use:
- *atonic wounds*, ulcers, burns, fistula
- coryza, laryngitis, bronchitis, whooping cough

Methods of use:

Internal:
- essence: 2 or 3 drops in honey water.
- *gomenol oil* at 50%, in capsules of 0.25g (2 to 10 a day, progressively), or 5 to 20 drops in an infusion.
- in hypodermic injections (in oily solution at 20%, 10 to 20cc average: Couvreur).

External:
- oily solution at 5 to 10% on dressings (burns, ulcers).
- *gomenol water*, at 2 to 5 parts per thousand, in compresses and washes of all kinds.
- *ephedrinised oil compound:*

  ephedrin base 0.30g
  essence of niaouli 1.50g
  olive oil 30cc

  2 or 3 drops in each nostril, 3 times a day.

N.B.
1. *Gomenol* (named after Gomen in New Caledonia) is an essence of niaouli purified of its irritant aldehydes. The local inhabitants have long used it to purify water.
2. The essence neutralises the tuberculosis bacillus at a dose of 0.4%.

Nutmeg

Myristica fragrans

Myristicaceae

This is the kernel of the fruit of the nutmeg tree, a tree which can grow to a height of 45 feet, producing, over a period of 10–30 years, between 1,500 and 2,000 nuts annually. The trees are male or female (one male tree can fertilise 20 female trees). The stone of the fruit is enclosed within a husk which, when dried, is known as *mace*.

Areas of production:
tropical countries, the Moluccas, the Antilles, Sumatra, Java, India.

Parts used:
powder and essence obtained by steam distillation of the kernel. The liquid essence, which has a distinctive odour and sharp, pungent taste, is aromatic when diluted. (An aromatic essence is also extracted from mace).

Principal known constituents:
"nutmeg butter", a fixed oil obtained by hot-pressing the kernels, contains myristine, butyrin, olein, palmitine and stearine. The essence contains 80% pinene and camphene, 8% dipentene, 6% terpenic alcohols (linalol, borneol, terpineol, geraniol), 4% myristicine and various substances such as eugenol and safrol.

Properties:
Internal use:
- general and intestinal antiseptic
- carminative
- digestive stimulant
- general, cerebral and circulatory stimulant
- dissolvent of gallstones (?)
- emmenagogue

External use:
- analgesic

Indications:
Internal use:
- intestinal infections
- chronic diarrhoea
- digestive problems (aids digestion of mutton and starchy foods (Leclerc))

161

- bad breath ("nutmeg sweetens the breath and corrects halitosis": John Gerard)
- loss of appetite
- flatulence
- debility
- gallstones
- scanty periods

External use:
- rheumatic pains
- toothache

Methods of use:
Internal:
- in food
- essence: 2 or 3 drops, 2 to 3 times a day in honey water or in an alcoholic solution; or in an infusion (Leclerc):

    essential oil of mace .... 25 drops
    granulated sugar 40g

    ½ a teaspoon of this sweetened oil dissolved in a glass of hot water.

External:
- "nutmeg butter" in liniments for the treatment of rheumatic pains and toothache.
- *nerve balm*, used in the treatment of rheumatic pains, is a mixture of the essences of rosemary and clove together with nutmeg butter.

N.B.
1. In high doses (7–12g) the essence has as stupefacient effect and acts as a circulatory sedative (Cadéac and Meunier). The symptoms of poisoning are similar to those of extreme alcoholic intoxication (delirium, hallucinations, stupor, loss of consciousness).
2. The essence is an ingredient of certain aromatic spirits, compound balm and various apéritifs and liqueurs, e.g. vermouth, raspail, *génépi*. Essence of mace is also used in certain drinks.
3. See under *Cinnamon* for the formulae for Italian essence and "Parfait amour", an aphrodisiac liqueur. See under *Rosemary* for the formula for an aphrodisiac bath.

Onion[1]

Allisum cepa

Liliaceae

The diuretic, tonic and antiseptic properties of the onion have been recognised since antiquity (Dioscorides, Pliny). It promotes health and longevity. Among the Bulgarians, who are great onion-eaters, may be counted many centenarians.

Parts used:
the bulb and its juice.

Principal known constituents:
sugar, vitamins A, B and C, mineral salts: sodium, potassium, calcareous phosphate and nitrate, iron, sulphur, iodine, silica, phosphoric and acetic acids, allyl disulphide, propyl disulphide, volatile oil, glucokinine, oxidase, diastase (these last two constituents are sterilised by heat).

Properties
Internal use:
- *general stimulant* (hepatic, renal and of the nervous system)
- *powerful diuretic* (dissolving and eliminating urea and chlorides)
- antirheumatic
- *antiscorbutic*
- antiseptic and *anti-infection* (antistaphylococcic: the onion acts in this respect like an antibiotic (Binet))
- secretary, expectorant
- digestive stimulant (aids digestion of farinaceous foods)
- *controls glandular balance*
- antisclerotic, antithrombosis
- aphrodisiac (early studies in this have been revived by H. Hull Walton)
- *hypoglycaemic*
- antiscrofulous
- vermifuge
- mild hypnotic
- curative for the skin and hair

1   Although it is included in this volume on account of its essence, I have in fact never prescribed onion in the form of its essential oil, for two reasons: first, because the onion is effective in its original form, and secondly because the odour of onion essence (like garlic) is one of the most unpleasant.

External use:
- emollient and resolvent
- antiseptic
- analgesic
- mosquito repellent

Indications:
Internal use:
- *debility*, physical and mental strain, growing pains
- *oliguria, retention of fluid* (oedema, ascites, pleurisy, pericarditis)
- *dropsy*
- *azotaemia, chloraemia*
- rheumatism, arthritis
- gallstones
- *intestinal fermentation* (*diarrhoea*)
- *genito-urinary infections*
- respiratory diseases (colds, bronchitis, asthma, laryngitis)
- influenza
- sluggish digestion
- *glandular disorders*
- puberty
- obesity
- arteriosclerosis, prevention of thrombosis
- *retarding senescence*
- *prostatism*, enlargement of prostate
- impotence
- *diabetes*
- adenitis, *lymphatism, rickets*
- intestinal parasites

External use:
- abscesses (hot), whitlows, boils, wasp stings
- haemorrhoids
- chilblains, chapped skin
- migraine
- cerebral congestion, meningitis
- deafness, buzzing in the ears
- toothache
- verrucas, warts
- sores, ulcers, burns
- freckles, alopecia
- mosquitoes (to repel)

Methods of use:
Internal:
1. – *onion* eaten raw or marinated for a few hours in olive oil. In salads, hors-d'oeuvre and *all* soups.

- chopped finely and taken in milk or stock, or spread on a slice of bread with butter or dripping.
- one chopped onion, steeped for a few hours in hot water. Drink this mixture in the morning before breakfast with a few drops of lemon juice.
- against *influenza*: leave 2 minced onions to steep in $\frac{1}{2}$ a litre of water. 1 glass of the maceration between meals and 1 at bedtime, for a fortnight.
- against *diarrhoea*: a handful of onion peelings to a litre of water. Boil for 10 minutes. Drink $\frac{1}{2}$ a litre a day
- against *diarrhoea in infants*: infuse 3 chopped onions in a litre of boiling water for 2 hours. Sweeten.
- against *intestinal parasites*: leave one large onion (minced) to steep for 6 days in a litre of white wine. 1 glass first thing each morning for a week when the moon is on the wane. Repeat for 2 or 3 months.
- against *rheumatism*: a decoction of 3 chopped unpeeled onions to 1 litre of water. Boil for 15 minutes and strain. Drink 1 glass on rising and 1 at bedtime.
- against *gallstones*: brown one large onion, finely chopped, in 4 tablespoonsful of olive oil. Add 150g water and 40g unsalted lard. Boil for 10 minutes. Drink very hot on several evenings in succession. 2 hours later, at bedtime, drink 1 cup of a decoction of black alder (*Frangula*) (2 to 5g of dried bark to 1 cup of water. Bring to the boil then remove from heat and allow to infuse for 4 to 6 hours until cold). This treatment should be given once a year.

2. – *Alcoholic tincture*: marinate fresh onion in an equal weight of 90° alcohol for 10 days. 3 to 5 teaspoons a day (1 teaspoon = 5g onion).

3. – 20% spirits: 5 to 10g twice a day at meals, in sugared water.

4. – *Wine* (P. Carles):

    onion finely chopped............................. 300g
    clear honey 100g
    white wine 600g

Leave to steep for 48 hours. Strain, 2 to 4 tablespoonsful a day (50g = 15g onion).

External:
- mustard plasters with raw onion (as with garlic) to treat *rheumatism*.
- *against cerebral congestion, meningitis*: treatment of choice, rub the temples with an onion, and pack the feet in 1 to 2kg of chopped onions (leave for 8 to 10 hours).
- against *migraine*: poultices of raw onions applied to the forehead.
- against *retention of urine, oliguria*: poultices of raw onion applied to the abdomen.

- against *warts, verrucas*: a mixture of onion, sea salt and clay in equal parts. Or hollow out an onion and fill with coarse salt and rub the wart morning and night with the liquid so obtained. Or rub the wart with half a red onion.
- against *wasp stings and insect bites*: rub the affected area for 1 to 2 minutes with a piece of onion (do not forget to remove the sting).
- against *abscesses, boils, haemorrhoids*: apply poultices of cooked onions. One onion, *baked in the oven and applied hot* brings abscesses, phlegmons and boils to a head.
- for *whitlows*: cover with a piece of onion peeling.
- for *chilblains, chapped skin, grazes*: apply compresses of onion juice.
- for *wounds, sores, cuts, ulcers* and *burns*: the fine membrane separating each layer of an onion can be used as an antiseptic dressing. Apply to the affected part, cover with gauze and complete the dressing.
- against *freckles*[1]: rub with vinegar in which crushed onions have been macerated; or rub with onion juice.
- against *buzzing in the ears*: earplugs of cotton-wool soaked in onion juice.
- against *deafness*: mix 30g of onion juice and 30g of spirits, and heat. Place 3 or 4 drops in the ear 3 times a day including once at bedtime.
- against *toothache*: apply a wad of cotton-wool soaked in onion juice to the cavity.
- one onion cut in half and put beside the bed will repel mosquitoes.

N.B.
1. Onion is *hypoglycaemic* because of its glucokinine content (J. P. Collip, 1923 and Laurin's experiments on rabbits in 1934, using subcutaneous injections of aqueous extracts. It is slower to take effect than insulin, but its effects are longer-lasting).
2. Raw onion has an elective effect on the urinary system, cooked onion on the digestive system.
3. *Spring onion treatment* is indicated as similar in effect to dandelion, grape or mineral water treatments. The shoots of young onions can also be eaten in spring (raw or in soups).
4. Onion soup is a marvellous cure for digestive troubles and flatulence, as well as the 'morning after'! (Brown the onions before eating).
5. Against *colds*: onion syrup. Slice the onions in rings, put on a plate and sprinkle with sugar. Leave to macerate for 24 hours. 2 to 5 tablespoons a day (Marcel Morlet).

1 Another recommend treatment (which I have not tried, but which has the advantage of a pleasant odour) is *benzoin skin lotion*: 10g tincture of benzoin in ½ a litre rosewater. This preparation may be used in everyday skincare.

6. Against *dropsy*, the following treatment is recommended: an exclusive diet of bread and milk 3 times a day with the addition of chopped raw onion. An improvement in the patient's condition becomes apparent after about a week. After 2 weeks profuse urination will occur.
7. Cut in two and inhaled deeply, an onion can stop a nervous attack.
8. An onion baked in the oven and applied to the soles of the feet at bedtime can be beneficial to asthmatic and cardiac sufferers.
9. Onion juice was highly recommended by the Salerno School as a cure for alopecia. Arab doctors prescribed a mixture of onion, salt and pepper applied locally as a cure for hair loss.
10. In 1972, Professor N. Kharchenko, head of the Department of Pharmacology at the Medical Institute of Kharkov, published the results of *ten years' study* of the onion. His findings include in particular:
    – Vitamins C, B, carotene, antibiotics;
    – digestive, anti-atherosclerotic, anticholesteric, hypotensive and cardiotonic properties (both curative and preventive);
    – fresh onion juice destroys the diphtheria and tuberculosis bacilli;
    – indicated for tonsillitis, influenza and pulmonary infections;
    – in *external use*, fresh onion juice to be used on suppurating and infected wounds;
    – a glycerine-based preparation is an effective treatment for Trichomonas cervicitis (a gynaecological disorder).
    "Essential," the author writes, "to the diet, especially of elderly people, the onion is also a very inexpensive medicine which retains its therapeutic properties over a long period."
11. To purify the breath after eating onion: chew 2 or 3 coffee beans, a few sprigs of parsley, or an apple; or rinse out the mouth with spirits of mint. To remove the smell from the hands: rub them in salted water or water to which ammonia has been added (2 tablespoonsful to a litre of tepid water).
12. It is said that when the layers of skin round onions are thick and numerous, the winter will be severe.

Some useful hints:
1. To remove fingermarks from doors and windows, rub them with the cut surface of an onion (or a potato).
2. To exterminate woodworm: rub the affected areas every day for 10 to 15 days with a halved onion.
3. To protect brasses from fly stains, brush them over with onion juice.
4. To preserve stoves and nickel objects from rust, rub with a piece of onion.
5. To clean brasses: a mixture of moist earth and crushed onion is excellent.

6. To clean windows and knives – even slightly rusty – use a piece of onion.
7. To restore the shine to patent leather belts and bags, rub them with a piece of onion.
8. Onion juice can be used as invisible ink – the writing becomes visible when the paper is exposed to heat.

Orange Blossom

Citrus aurantium

Rutaceae

Also known as Seville orange, bigarade, sour orange, *Citrus bigaradia*.

Its origin in China, it is now grown in the Midi region of France, southern Italy, Sicily, Algeria, the Iberian Peninsula, Mexico, California, South America and the countries bordering the Indian Ocean.

Cultivation has produced the *Citrus sinensis*, or sweet orange.

Parts used:

essence of orange flowers (or *neroli*), obtained by steam distillation of fresh flowers. One tonne of flowers will yield approximately 1kg of essence (some trees will produce 30kg of flowers a year).

Principal known constituents:

30% linalol, geraniol, nerol, benzoic, anthranylic and phenylacetic esters, traces of indole and jasmone.

Properties:
Internal use:
- diminishes cardiac contractions
- dulls nervous sensibility, sedative
- lightly hypnotic

Indications:
- cardiac spasm, palpitations, false angina pectoris
- chronic diarrhoea, nervous dyspepsia
- insomnia

Method of use:
- 1 to 3 drops several times a day in honey water.

N.B.
1. Distilled orange-flower water is made from the blossom.
2. From the peel, which is inedible, is derived the *essence of bitter oranges*.
3. *Portugal essence* is produced from the *sweet* orange tree.

Origanum

Origanum vulgare

Labiatea

(Origanum floribundum, Origanum glandulosum, North African species).

Origanum vulgare is also known as oregano, wild marjoram, joy of the mountain.

Parts used:
flowering tops, essence.

Principal known constituents:
essential oil (thymol and carvacrol), gum, resin.

Properties:
Internal use:
- *antispasmodic sedative*
- apéritif
- *stomachic*
- *carminative*
- *expectorant* (thins bronchial secretions)
- *antiseptic* to the respiratory tract
- emmenagogue
- antirheumatic

External use:
- parasiticide
- analgesic

Indications:
Internal use:
- loss of appetite
- gastric atony (sluggish digestion)
- *aerophagy*, distension, particularly in psychopaths (imaginary or mental diseases)
- chronic *bronchitis, tickling cough, whooping cough*
- pulmonary *tuberculosis*
- *asthma*
- acute or chronic rheumatism, muscular rheumatism
- *absence of menstrual periods* (outside pregnancy)

External use:
- lice

170

- rheumatism of muscles and joints
- cellulitis

Methods of use:
Internal:
- infusion: 1 dessertspoonful in a cup of boiling water. Infuse for 10 minutes. Take 1 cup before, during or after each meal.
- essence: 3 to 5 drops in honey water 2 to 4 times a day.
- fluid extract: 3 to 5g a day (divide the dose).

External:
- poultices, covered with a hot bran or linseed meal poultice (rheumatic or muscular pain)
- *antirheumatic liniment*:

> essence of origanum............................... 5g
> spirit of rosemary 95g

applied in friction rubs to the affected parts.

- *anticellulite ointment*:

> alcoholic tincture – or fluid extract – of climbing ivy ... 5g
> essence of origanum......................... 20 drops
> lanolin 20g
> lard or vaseline 40g

This may be used in the treatment of *cellulitis*, or as an *antirheumatic ointment*.

- *ointment to treat lice* (Renaudet, 1913):

> essence of origanum.............................
> essence of lemongrass......................... } 15 drops of each
> essence of thyme.............................
> essence of geranium ....
> melted clear wax.............................. 5g
> vaseline 85g

N.B.
See under *Rosemary* for the formula for an aphrodisiac bath.

Peppermint

Mentha piperita

Labiatae

An indigenous plant, now cultivated, probably derived from a hybrid of *Mentha viridis* (spearmint). Widely grown in England, France, Italy and America.

Both the leaves and essence are used, the latter obtained by steam distillation of leaves and flowering tops.

Principal known constituents:
chiefly, an *essence* (2 to 3%) which contains from 30 to 70% menthol, terpenes (menthene, phellandrene, limonene), a ketone (menthone) and tannin.

A better quality essence is found in the plants of colder countries, for instance the Mitcham variety in England.

Properties:
Internal use:
 – *stimulant* of the nervous system, general tonic
 – *stomachic*
 – *antispasmodic,* (gastric spasm, colic)
 – *carminative*
 – general *antiseptic*, especially intestinal
 – emmenagogue
 – expectorant
 – vermifuge
 – slight aphrodisiac
 – anti-galactagogue
 – in strong doses, prevents sleep

External use:
 – antiseptic
 – parasiticide
 – antispasmodic
 – analgesic
 – insect repellent (mosquitos, gnats)

Indications:
Internal use:
 – general fatigue
 – *sluggish digestion*, indigestion
 – gastralgia
 – *aerophagy* (Martial)
 – gastric spasm and colic (Trousseau)

- *flatulence*, diarrhoea, cholera
- gastro-intestinal poisoning
- bad breath (due to dyspepsia)
- liver complaints
- nervous vomiting (Trousseau)
- *palpitations, vertigo*
- migraine, tremors, paralysis
- scanty or painful menstrual periods
- impotence
- asthma, chronic bronchitis (aids expectoration)
- tuberculosis
- intestinal parasites

External use:
- scabies
- asthma, bronchitis, sinusitis
- migraine, toothache
- repels mosquitos, gnats

Methods of use:
Internal:
- infusion: 1 dessertspoonful of leaves to a cup of boiling water. 3 cups a day, after or between meals (warning with regard to individual susceptibilities – can inhibit sleep).
- spirit: 15 to 20 drops in a glass of sweetened water.
- syrup: 20 to 100g a day.
- essence: 2 to 5 drops several times a day, either in a draught or in honey water (take every 5 minutes during spasm).
- *stimulant elixir:*

      spirits of mint 20g
      sugar syrup 100g
      cinnamon water 50g
  to be taken by the teaspoon or tablespoon.

- *stomachic potion:.*

      spirits of mint 15g
      spirits of aniseed 15g
      cinnamon syrup 30g
      lime-blossom water 120g
  to be taken by the teaspoon or tablespoon.

External:
- in inhalations (for asthma, bronchitis, sinusitis).
- in oils for the relief of *migraine* and toothache.
- in the treatment of scabies: see under *Lavender* (Helmerich's ointment).
- to repel mosquitos: put a few drops of peppermint on the pillow at night.
- essence of peppermint is used in toothpaste and various mouthwashes. Its antispasmodic effect is made use of in certain purgatives.

N.B.
1. Mint leaves make a delicious and beneficial addition to any salad.
2. A decoction of Corsican moss in which a few mint-leaves have been infused is one of the *best vermifuges* for children.
3. To restore the menstrual cycle: a pinch each of the leaves of wild mint, rosemary, wormwood and sage. Infuse (without heat) for 8 days in 2 litres of red wine. Strain. Take a glass first thing in the morning for ten days.
4. Essence of peppermint kills staphylococcus in $3\frac{1}{2}$ hours (L. Sévelinges). It will neutralise the tuberculosis bacillus at a dose of 0.4% (Courmont, Morel, Rochaix)..
5. See under *Clove* for the formula for an aromatic dentifrice.
   See under *Rosemary* for the formula for an aphrodisiac bath.
6. *Alternative formula for an aromatic dentifrice.*

spirits of guaiacum	187g
spirits of camphor	4g
essence of peppermint	6 drops
essence of cochlearia	6 drops
essence of rosemary	6 drops

7. An infusion of peppermint taken at night can inhibit sleep; some people use it specifically for this purpose.

Other varieties of Mint
1. JAPANESE MINT (a variety of FIELD MINT) *(Mentha arvensis var. piperascens)*. Its essence contains 75% menthol; it is the principal source of essence and of menthol, providing over $\frac{3}{4}$ of the total world production.
2. CURLY MINT *(M. spicata var. crispa)*, SPEARMINT *(M. viridis)*, WATER MINT, etc.

Pine

Pinus sylvestris

Pinaceae

Also known as Scots pine. Found extensively in the cold upland regions of Europe, Scandinavia and the USSR, indigenous to these areas.

Parts used: the buds, the thick distilled resin of the tree (turpentine) and the essential oil obtained by steam distillation of the *needles.*

Principal known constituents: essence of turpentine (pinene, camphene, terpenes, etc), mallol, essential oil: pinene, sylvestrene, bornyl acetate, cadinene, pumilone. The buds contain more than 200g of resin per kilo.

Properties:
 Internal use:
 − Powerful antiseptic of the *respiratory tract*, balsamic
 − antiseptic of the *urinary and hepatic systems*
 − *stimulant of the adrenal cortex*

External use:
 − rubefacient (rheumatic complaints)
 − antiseptic balsam

Indications:
 Internal use:
 − *all infections of the respiratory tract* (colds, bronchitis, tracheitis, pneumonia, asthma, tuberculosis, etc)
 − influenza
 − *urinary infections* (pyelitis, cystitis, prostatitis)
 − cholecystitis (inflammation of the gall-bladder)
 − *infections in general*
 − *gallstones*
 − *impotence*
 − rickets
 − gastralgia, intestinal pains

External use:
 − pulmonary diseases
 − influenza, sinusitis
 − rheumatism, gout (baths)
 − excessive sweating of the feet
 − scabies, lice

Methods of use:

Internal:
- *infusion:* of the buds, 20 to 50g to 1 litre of water. 3 cups a day.
- syrup, of the buds: 50 to 100g a day.
- tincture: 10 to 20 drops, twice or three times daily.
- *essential oil:* 3 to 5 drops in honey water 3 or 4 times daily; alternatively in alcoholic suspension.

External:
- *inhalations of the essential oil* (influenza, sinusitis, bronchitis):
- *a mixture for inhalation:*

essential oil of lavender	1g
essential oil of pine	2g
essential oil of thyme	2g
essential oil of eucalyptus	4g
90° alcohol	150cc

   One dessertspoonful or tablespoonful to a bowl of boiling water. Inhale 2 or 3 times daily for 8–15 days.
- essence or buds, in *baths*: local bathing for dyshidrosis and for excessive sweating of the feet, general baths for rheumatism and gout. Also aids expectoration by loosening phlegm.

N.B.
1. See under *Cinnamon* for a formula to treat lice and scabies.
2. The cluster pine *(Pinus maritima* or *P. pinaster*) yields Bordeaux turpentine, galipot, essence of turpentine, pine pitch and wood tar, etc.
3. The silver fir (*Abies pectinata* or *alba*) yields Strassburg or Vosges turpentine.
4. In 1534 Jacques Cartier learned from the North American Indians the antiscorbutic properties of the extract of pine-needles.

Rosemary

Rosmarinus officinalis

Labiatae

Common in the South of France (Provence), Italy, Spain, Tunisia, Dalmatia.

Rosemary is used in cooking, in infusions (the flowering tops and leaves) or as an essential oil obtained by steam distillation of the flowering tops (100kg of plants provide approximately 1.5kg of essence).

Principal known constituents: essential oil: pinene, camphene, cineol, borneols (15%), camphors, resin, a bitter principle, saponin.

Properties:
Internal use:
- *general stimulant* (similar to peppermint, melissa, sage, thyme) and *cardiotonic,*
- *stimulant of the adrenal cortex* restorative
- hypertensive (Caujolle, Cazal)
- stomachic
- *pulmonary antiseptic,* antitussive
- antidiarrhoeic, intestinal antiseptic
- carminative
- antirheumatic, antineuralgic
- *antigout*
- *cholagogue choleretic* (in animals an intra-venous infusion doubles the volume of bile secreted: Chabrol. Parturier's and Rousselle's experiments with duodenal intubation)
- *emmenagogue*
- cerebral stimulant
- diuretic, sudorific

External use:
- cicatrising (wounds, burns), resolvent
- parasiticide
- aphrodisiac

Indications:
Internal use:
- *general debility*
- physical and mental strain *(loss of memory)*
- hypotension (low blood pressure)
- impotence
- *chlorosis,* adenitis, lymphatism (glandular disorders)

- asthma, chronic bronchitis, whooping cough, influenza
- intestinal infections, colitis, diarrhoea
- flatulence, halitosis
- *disorders of the liver, cholecystitis, jaundice* from hepatitis or from obstruction, *cirrhosis, gallstones*
- hypercholesterolaemia (excess of cholesterol in the blood)
- *atonic dyspepsia* (painful digestion), gastric pains, constipation
- rheumatism, gout
- dysmenorrhoea (painful periods), leucorrhoea
- *migraine*
- disorders of the nervous system: hysteria, *epilepsy, the after-effects of paralysis*, weakness of the limbs
- cardiac complaints of nervous origin, palpitations
- *vertigo*, fainting

External use:
- wounds, sores, burns
- rheumatism
- muscular pains, stiffness
- leucorrhoea
- lice, scabies
- general fatigue, weakness in children, poor eyesight (baths)

Methods of use:
Internal:
- *infusion* (leaves or flowers); 1 dessertspoon to a cup of boiling water. Leave to infuse for 10 minutes. 1 cup before or after meals.
- *fluid extract:* 3 to 5g a day.
- *essential oil* 3 or 4 drops twice or three times daily, in alcoholic solution or in honey water.

External:
- in *compresses*, for *rheumatism*: a decoction using a handful to a litre of water. Boil for 10 minutes. The same decoction may be used in vaginal douches (leucorrhoea) and in lotions for sores, minor wounds.
- in *friction rubs* with an alcoholic solution of the essence at 2% (rheumatism).
- essence of rosemary plus olive oil, in friction rubs for muscular pain
- *antirheumatic liniment:*

      tincture of ginger................................. 40g
      essence of origanum.............................. 2g
      spirit of rosemary 60g
   in friction rubs.
- see under *Ginger* for my own formula.

– in *fortifying baths* (especially for children), and in the treatment of rheumatism and weak eyesight. Preferably morning baths.

– *aphrodisiac bath:*

crushed nutmeg.	50g
rosemary	⎫
sage	⎪
origanum	⎬ 500g of each
mint	⎪
camomile flowers	⎪
boiling water	⎭

Leave to infuse for 12 hours, then add:

tincture of juniper.	100g
tincture of clove	100g

for a deep bath.

– scabies, lice: see under *Cinnamon* for the formula (an infusion of the leaves and flowers in spirits of wine has always been a recommended treatment for scabies).

N.B.

1. Essence of rosemary in an excessive quantity has a strong tendency to induce epilepsy and, like fennel essence, will make animals timid and apprehensive. The essences of sage, wormwood and hyssop, on the other hand, though equally liable to induce epilepsy, cause animals to become aggressive.

2. The spirit of rosemary (the elixir of youth was reputedly obtained by distilling cedar, rosemary and turpentine) used to carry the name "Water of the Queen of Hungary" (1370). It is supposed to have transformed a paralytic, gout-ridden septuagenarian princess into a seductive girl whose hand was sought in marriage by a king of Poland.

3. Rosemary was an ingredient of "Vinegar of the Four Thieves" (Marseilles vinegar). It is a constituent of aromatic wine, soothing balms, Dardel water (a stimulant), the vulnerary spirit listed in the Codex (for contusion), nerve balm (stimulant, antirheumatic), rosemary ointment (lice) and veterinary ointments.

4. See under *Peppermint* for a formula for a dentifrice elixir.

Sage

Salvia officinalis

Labiatae

A common garden plant, grown throughout the world. The Romans called it *herba sacra*. For the Salerno School, it was "Salvia salvatrix, natura conciliatrix". It has always been widely used as a popular remedy and is one of the best-known medicinal plants. There are roughly 500 varieties of sage.

Parts used: leaves, flowers, essential oil (which can bring on epileptic fits and have a toxic effect on the nervous system).

Principal known constituents: tannin, an oestrogenic principle, an essence: borneol, salviol, (or camphor of sage), cineol, salvene, thujone (a ketone, about 50%).

Properties:
Internal use:
- *tonic*, general stimulant (activates the *nervous system* and the adrenal cortex)
- regulates the balance of the nerves and the parasympathetic system
- *antispasmodic*, calmative
- apéritif
- *antiseptic*
- *antisudorific* (Van Swieten)
- depurative
- *diuretic*
- *hypertensive* (Caujolle, Cazel)
- *emmenagogue* (the purified extract of sage, injected in mice, causes reactions similar to those which folliculin produces: Kroszcynski and Bychowska)
- conducive of conception
- anticancer (?)
- anti-galactagogue

External use:
- astringent
- healing (cicatrasing)
- antiseptic
- tonic, antirheumatic (baths)

Indications:
Internal use:
- has a restorative effect on the whole body; indicated for all kinds of

illness: for the digestive organs and the liver, for urinary, pulmonary and pleural diseases, etc.
- *general debility* (convalescence), *nervous debility*
- *dyspepsia* due to gastro-intestinal atony, sluggish digestion, loss of appetite
- nervous afflictions: tremors, vertigo, paralysis
- apoplexy
- *asthma*, chronic bronchitis
- *night sweats in tuberculosis patients* and convalescents
- profuse sweating of hands and armpits
- adenitis, lymphatism (glandular disorders)
- intermittent fevers
- *oliguria* (insufficient urine)
- *hypotension* (low blood pressure)
- regulates erratic menstrual periods, *dysmenorrhoea* (painful periods)
- *menopause*
- *sterility* (Lyte)
- diarrhoea (in tuberculosis patients and babies)
- malignant conditions (?)
- ante-natal preparation
- to halt lactation

External use:
- leucorrhoea (vaginal douches)
- *thrush, stomatitis,* sore throat (angina, tonsillitis), laryngitis, tooth-ache
- care of gums, gingivitis
- asthma
- *atonic wounds,* sores, ulcers
- dermatosis (eczema)
- debility in children, rickets, scrofulosis
- alopecia
- wasp stings, insect bites
- domestic disinfectant

Contra-indication: breast-feeding

Methods of use.
Internal:
- *infusion:* 20g of flowers and leaves to 1 litre boiling water. Infuse for 10 minutes. 3 cups a day.
- *tincture:* 30 to 40 drops twice daily in a little hot water.
- *liquid extract* of stabilised sage: 1 teaspoon in an infusion of balm *(Melissa)* at night to restore *nervous equilibrium* and against night sweats.
- *essence:* 2 to 4 drops 3 times a day in alcoholic solution or in honey water.

181

- *powder:* 1 to 4g a day.
- *tonic wine:*

  sage leaves 80g
  wine (red or white) .... 1 litre

  Leave to macerate for a week. 1 to 3 tablespoons after meals. Recommended by Leclerc for debility, physical or mental exhaustion, nervous debility, dystonia of the autonomic nervous system, following prolonged illness (also in the case of intermittent fevers).
- used also in preparations for thrush.
- mulled wine with sage is an acceptable substitute for mulled wine with cinnamon.
- *antisudorific potion:*

  liquid extract of stabilised sage 50g
  orange-flower syrup 30g
  water 150cc

  1 tablespoon at bedtime *(tuberculosis, menopause).*

External:
- *emmenagogic suppositories:*

  liquid extract of stabilised sage 0.25g
  balm of poplar 1g
  cocoa butter 3g
  white wax .... sufficient for 1 suppository

  1 or 2 a day (amenorrhoea, dysmenorrhoea, *sterility?).*
- *decoction:* a handful of leaves and flowers to a litre of water. Boil for 10 minutes.

  use as *mouthwash* (for *thrush*, stomatitis, mouth ulcers).

  use in *vaginal douches* (leucorrhoea), use in *compresses* on leg ulcers, atonic wounds and sores, dermatosis, eczema.
- *tincture:* with rum in equal parts: in friction rubs for *alopecia.*
- against insect bites, wasp stings: apply crushed sage leaves.
- the dried leaves may be smoked in cases of asthma – see Chapter 6 for recipe.
- *ointment* with:

  sage leaves 30g
  ground ivy leaves 30g
  lard 250g
  white wax 45g

  Cook all the ingredients together and remove the plants (for atonic wounds and sores, ulcers, bruising).
- baths of the infusion: for debility in children, rickets, scrofulosis, rheumatism
- see under *Rosemary* for the formula for an aphrodisiac bath.

N.B.
1. An infusion of sage taken regularly for a month before childbirth will considerably reduce labour pains.

2. Meadow clary or meadow sage *(Salvia pratensis)* has the same properties as *S. officinalis*, but to a lesser degree. Clary *(Salvia sclarea)* also shares the same properties. It is used particularly for its stimulant and emmenagogic properties (to treat amenorrhoea and dysmenorrhoea) and its leaves are still used today in the treatment of whooping cough. Its essence contains sclareol; it is used in cosmetics for its scent of ambergris and as a base for perfumes. According to Elt Muller, this variety of sage was used in the past by German wine-merchants to disguise their products. An infusion of clary and elder would give the agreeable bouquet of a muscat wine to Rhine wines, and this is undoubtedly why the plant is called in Germany *Muskateller Salbei*.
3. To disinfect sickrooms after serious illnesses, burn sage leaves over charcoal.
4. To make the provençal soup *Aigo-bouido*, infuse a dozen sage leaves, together with salt, pepper, garlic and 100g of olive oil, in 2 litres of water. Boil for 10 minutes and pour over slices of bread.

Sandalwood

Santalum album, Santalum spicatum

Santalaceae

A tree from the East Indies and Australia (parasitic: its roots bury themselves in those of neighbouring trees).

The *wood* itself is used, and in particular the *essence* obtained from it by steam distillation.

Principal known constituents: the essence, containing 80% terpenic alcohols calculated as santalol; fusanols, santalic and teresantalic acids, carbides.

Properties:
Internal use:
- *antiseptic (urinary* and pulmonary)
- tonic and aphrodisiac
- astringent (the wood)

Indications:
- *specific for infections of the urinary tract:* gonorrhhoea, cystitis, colibacillosis
- impotence
- chronic bronchitis
- obstinate diarrhoea (the wood)

Methods of use:
- capsules of the essence at 0.25g (5 drops): 4 to 20 a day *(S. album)*; 6 to 12 a day *(S. spicatum)*.
- santalol: capsules at 0.50g; 2 to 4 a day between meals.
- in high doses: feeling of heat in the pit of the stomach, extreme thirst and sometimes nausea.

N.B.
1. *Santalum album* is the white sandalwood. *Santalum spicatum* is the Australian sandal.
2. In the old days, sandalwood was used for making furniture and decorating temples on account of its scent and its resistance to attack by insects. In powdered form it was burned during religious ceremonies. It is highly valued in the East as a perfume.

Savory

Satureia montana

Labiatae

Also known as Winter Savory.

Savory enjoyed great prestige in antiquity. it is always included as an ingredient in many digestive liqueurs and certain healing remedies.

Parts used: the whole plant, the flowering tops, the essence.

Used in the kitchen for its aromatic and antitoxic qualities (it is said to be one of the best seasonings for gamy meat), it is universally included in the preparation of raw vegetables, starchy cooked dishes and, with sage, tomato sauces.

The *essence* is obtained by distillation, it contains pinene, carvacrol (up to 30 to 40 %), cymene (20 to 25%), terpenes (40 to 50%), cineol, a small amount of thymol.

Properties:

Internal use:
- digestive stimulant
- *stimulant* (especially *mental* and of the adrenal cortex)
- *aphrodisiac* (without too many expectations)
- antispasmodic
- carminative
- *antiseptic*, antiputrefactive
- vermifuge
- expectorant

External use:
- cicatrising (healing), resolvent

Indications:

Internal use:
- *painful digestion*, gastric atony
- *mental and sexual debility*
- gastric pains of nervous origin
- intestinal spasm
- flatulence, distension of the stomach
- intestinal parasites
- in Germany: all types of *diarrhoea*
- asthma, bronchitis

External use:
- sores

- insect bites
- deafness

Methods of use:
Internal:
- *Infusion* of the flowering tops: 5g to a cup of boiling water. Infuse for 10 minutes. 3 cups a day before or after meals.
- *essence:* 3 to 5 drops in honey water 2 or 3 times a day immediately after meals.

External:
- infusion of the whole plant: 25 to 30g to 1 litre of water. Use in lotions and compresses (for sores, wounds).
- to treat *deafness*: 3 or 4 drops of juice of savory in the ear, three times a day and again on retiring.

N.B.
1. In the old days a decoction of savory in wine was one of the medications used to treat mouth and throat ulcers, and toothache was relieved by rubbing the decayed tooth with savory essence while at the same time putting a drop in the ear.
2. *Satureia hortensis* (summer savory) has similar properties, but to a lesser degree.

New information
Although it is not included in the composition of pharmaceutical medicines, researchers at the Pharmacological Faculty at Montpellier have recently published an extremely interesting study on the antibacterial and antifungal powers of essence of savory. They compared it with other essences of the same family currently used in medicine: *Thymus vulgaris, Rosmarinus officinalis, Lavandula vera, Lavandula latifolia* and *Lavandin.*[1]

They were able to demonstrate the net superiority of the antimicrobial properties of essence of savory in respect of the microbe colonies they used: ten types of Staphylococcus, fourteen other micro-organisms and eleven funguses including *Candida albicans, C. tropicalis, Trichophyton interdigitalis.*

The essence of savory remained active at concentrations from 2 to 20 times weaker than the others. Only thyme produced equal results on more than one occasion, surpassing it in the case of *Candida pelliculosa.*

These facts are worth remembering in the treatment of numerous infections.

1 *Place de l'essence de Satureoa montana dans l'arsenal thérapeutique:* J. Pellecuer, Mme J. Allegrini, Mme Simeon de Buochberg and J. Passet (Lab. de Botanique et Cryptogamie du Pr. G. Privat, Fac. de Pharmacie de Montpellier), in *Plantes medicinales et Phytotherapie,* 1975, T. IX, No 2.

Tarragon

Artemisia dracunculus

Compositae

A pot-herb; a species of *Artemisia*; an excelllent seasoning which may be used, if the need arises, as a substitute for salt, pepper and vinegar.
The essence is obtained by distillation of the plant.

Principal known constituents: estragol (60–70%), 15 to 20% terpenes: ocimene, phellandrene.

Properties:
Internal use:
– *stimulant*, general and *digestive*
– apéritif
– stomachic
– *antispasmodic*
– internal antiseptic
– carminative
– emmenagogue
– vermifuge
– anticancer (?)

Indications:
– anorexia (loss of appetite)
– *dyspepsia*, sluggish digestion, gastralgia
– *intestinal spasm*, nervous dyspepsia
– *dystonia of the sympathetic nervous system*
– *hiccough*, aerophagy
– flatulence, putrefactive fermentations
– dysmenorrhoea (painful menstruation)
– intestinal *parasites*
– rheumatic pains
– malignant conditions (?)

Methods of use:
– in food (salads, preparations of raw vegetables, cooked dishes)
– infusion: 25 to 30g to a litre of water. Infuse for 10 minutes. After meals or during the course of the day.
– essence: 2 or 3 drops in an alcoholic solution or in honey water, 3 to 4 times a day.

N.B.
1. It is claimed by some that tarragon possesses anti-cancer properties.
2. People suffering from illnesses requiring a saltless diet will certainly benefit from using tarragon.
3. Against hiccoughs: chew a tarragon leaf or suck a sugar-lump impregnated with 3 or 4 drops of pure tarragon essence.

Terebinth

Essence of turpentine

The turpentines are resins extracted from certain species of conifers and *Anacardiaceae (Pinus laricio* or *nigra, Pinus maritima* or *pinaster, pinus sylvestris, Pinus palustris, Abies pectinata* or *alba, Pistachia terebinthus,* etc).

They are of a soft consistency and are formed by the dissolving of resinous principles in a mixture of liquid carbides.

They contain terpenes, mono and bicyclic carbides, acids and alcohols of high molecular weight.

The *essence* is obtained by distilling turpentine, especially common, or Bordeaux turpentine, with water or with water vapour which is not overheated. It has to be purified because it is viscous, coloured and acidic.

The *officinal essence* (recognised in the pharmacopoeia) is formed principally of invert turpentine. Together with water, and above all in the presence of air, if forms the hydrate *terpin* (which, in small doses, *loosens bronchial secretions* and is *diuretic*). Oxidising agents attack essence of turpentine with violence. The oxidised essence has oxidising properties identical to those of ozone.

Properties (some of which were known to Hippocrates, Dioscorides and Galen):
Internal use:
- *modifies tracheo-bronchial secretions* (phlegm), with beneficial effect
- *balsamic, pulmonary* and *genito-urinary antiseptic* (Richet and Héricaut) – antiseptic especially with regard to *Streptococcus*, given in the form of sub-cutaneous injections (as a terebinthinate artificial serum at a strength of 1/200) and intra-uterine and vaginal douches (emulsions of soap bark)
- haemostatic
- *dissolves gallstones*
- diuretic
- antispasmodic
- *antirheumatic*
- *vermifuge*
- *antidote to phosphorus*; particularly when old, the essence prevents the oxidisation of phosphorus.

External use:
- parasiticide
- analgesic
- revulsive (counter-irritant)
- antiseptic, cicatrising

Indications:
Internal use:
- *chronic* and fetid *bronchitis, pulmonary tuberculosis*
- urinary and renal infections, *cystitis,* urethritis
- leucorrhoea
- puerperal fever
- haemorrhage (intestinal, pulmonary, uterine; haemophilia, nose-bleeds)
- *gallstones*
- oliguria
- dropsy
- rheumatism
- spasms (colitis, whooping cough)
- flatulence
- migraine
- *intestinal parasites* (especially tapeworm)
- chronic constipation
- epilepsy
- *accidental consumption of phosphorus*

External use:
- *rheumatism, gout,* neuralgia, sciatica
- atonic wounds and sores, gangrenous wounds
- scabies, lice
- leucorrhoea, puerperal infections

Methods of use:
Internal:
- *essence* of turpentine is 4 times more active than turpentine itself. 1 to 4g a day in capsules or *perles* of 0.25g (4 to 16 capsules a day); or 6 to 10 drops in honey water, 3 or 4 times a day. *Children's dosage:* 0.20g a day for each year of age.
- *syrup:* 50 to 100g a day.
- *pills to treat kidney infections and cystitis:*

purified turpentine	10g
camphor	10g
extract of opium	1cg
extract of aconite	1cg

    Quantity for one pill. 3 or 4 a day.
- *pills for chronic bronchitis:*

purified turpentine	0.10g
benzoate of soda	0.10g

    Quantity for one pill. 5 to 10 a day.
- *syrup for chronic bronchitis:*

syrup of turpentine	
syrup of tar	50g of each
syrup of Tolu	
syrup of codeine	

    3 tablespoonfuls a day.

- *for gallstones: Durande's mixture:*

  officinal ether 20g

  essence of turpentine 10g

  15 to 30 drops a day.
- as an antidote to phosphorus: 5 to 15g in a resinous potion with carbonate of soda added. Then 2g a day for 4 to 5 days.
- *emulsion to counteract phosphorus poisoning:*

  essence of turpentine ..... ; .... 5 to 10g

  yolk of egg 1

  syrup of mint.................................... 50g

  water... 100g

  by the tablespoon, every 2 or 3 hours.

External:
- in inhalations:

  essence of turpentine 10g

  tincture of eucalyptus 30g

  tincture of benzoin 30g

  1 teaspoon to a bowl of boiling water.
- in liniments (atonic wounds and sores, gangrenous wounds, rheumatism, neuralgia). See under *Ginger* for an antirheumatic formula.

antirheumatic balm:

  balm of Fioravanti 250g

  soap 30g

  camphor.. 25g

  ammonia 8g

  essence of rosemary 6g

  essence of thyme............................... 2g

Use in friction rubs.

emulsion for baths:

  essence of turpentine 200g

  solution of coal-tar soap (1pt in 4)................ 200g

Shake well. Use half for a full bath. One or two tablespoons for local baths (the forearms). Against rheumatism.
- in subcutaneous injections (as a counter-irritant, to form fixation abscesses).
- in vaginal or intra-uterine douches:
- *emulsion for vaginal or intra-uterine douches:*

  essence of turpentine 250g

  tincture of quillaja 5g

  sterilised water 600g

Shake well. 2 tablespoons to a litre of boiling water (puerperal infection).
- parasiticide (fleas).

N.B.
Fioravanti's balm, often mentioned in studies on volatile oils, is a compound spirit of turpentine. It is obtained by distilling alcohol with turpentine, together with about 15 aromatic and resinous substances.

Thuja[1]

Thuja occidentalis

Coniferae

The "Arbor vitae", this tree originates from China and North America. It is cultivated in France. Its use in therapy was popularised by S. Hahnemann.

Parts used:
leaves, bark.

Principal known constituents:
a glucoside, an *essence* containing pinene, fenone and a convulsant ketone (thujone), tannins, etc.

Properties:
Internal use:
- expectorant
- mild *diuretic* and *urinary sedative*
- sudorific
- antirheumatic
- vermifuge
- anti-cancer (Ellingwood)

External use:
- tonic, local remedy

Indications:
Internal use:
- cystitis, *hypertrophy of the prostate*, pelvic congestion, incontinence (urinary) in plethoric women
- rheumatism
- intestinal parasites
- malignant conditions

External use:
- warts, verrucas, condylomas (syphylitic warts), polyps
- vegetations, (gargles)
- prophylactic of venereal diseases

1 Editor's Note: Thuja oil is a very poisonous essential oil and should only be used under strict medical supervision.

Methods of use:
Internal:
- leaves or bark: 10g to ½ a litre of water. Boil for 2 minutes. Infuse for 10 minutes. Drink within 24 hours.
- hydro-alcoholic extract: in pills at 0.10g (5 to 10 a day).
- tincture at 1 part in 5: 20 to 40 drops a day.
- essence: occasionally used as a vermifuge.

External:
- *essence* or *"mother-tincture"*: apply to the affected area with a cotton-wool pad twice daily, or in local injections (J. Sicard and P. Larue).

N.B.
Thuja is one of the constituents of Pfeiffer's *prophylactic soap*, which may be used to bathe the genitals immediately after suspected contact with venereal disease.
  Recommended by Pfeiffer against syphilitic infection.

Thyme

Thymus vulgaris

Labiatae

(Wild Thyme, or Mother of thyme, (*Thymus serpyllum*) can be used in the same way as *T. vulgaris* to treat the complaints listed below).

Thyme is one of the herbs especially blessed with a large number of therapeutic properties. It is used in the form of infusions (leaves and flowering tops) and its essential oil (obtained from the flowering tops by steam distillation) which is *redistilled* to eliminate irritant substances.

Principal known constituents:
tannin, bitter principle, essence containing 2 phenols (up to 60% thymol and carvacrol), terpenes: terpinene, cymene; alcohols: borneol, linalol.

Properties:
Internal use:
– *general stimulant*, physical and mental stimulant, stimulant of the capillary circulation
– nerve tonic
– said to stimulate the intelligence
– claimed to be *aphrodisiac*
– apéritif
– hypertensive (Caujolle, Cazal)
– *antispasmodic*
– stomachic
– *balsamic*, expectorant (modifies bronchial secretions)
– *antiseptic*: *intestinal*, *pulmonary*, genito-urinary
– stimulates production of white corpuscles in infectious diseases (leucocytosis)
– diuretic
– sudorific
– *emmenagogue*
– carminative
– *vermifuge*
– mild hypnotic

External use:
– *antiseptic* and bactericide (especially the peroxidised essence)
– *antivenomous*
– antiputretactive
– cicatrising
– *revulsive* (counter-irritant)
– antirheumatic
– *parasiticide*

Indications:
Internal use:
- *physical and mental debility*, anxiety, nervous debility, nervous deficiency, depressive states
- anaemia (in children)
- hypotension
- chlorosis
- *convulsive cough* (whooping cough: H. Schulz)
- *pulmonary diseases*: emphysema, mycosis, bronchitis
- tuberculosis
- *asthma*
- digestive atony (sluggish digestion)
- *intestinal infections* (typhoid), *urinary infections* (pyelitis)
- flatulence
- *illnesses resulting from chill* (influenza, head colds, stiffness, rigor, tonsillitis, sore throat): *one of the best remedies*
- *infectious diseases*
- furunculosis
- rheumatism
- circulatory disorders
- *abnormal cessation of menstrual periods*
- leucorrhoea (Girault, Dijon)
- *intestinal parasites* (roundworm, threadworm, hookworm, *tapeworm*)
- insomnia

External use:
- *dermatosis*, boils, sores
- leucorrhoea
- dental and oral hygiene ·
- general fatigue (baths)
- rheumatism of the joints and muscles, gout, arthritis
- hair loss
- influenza, bronchitis, sinusitis (see Pine)
- skin antiseptic
- lice, scabies
- insect bites, snake bites

Methods of use:
Internal:
- *infusion*: one sprig per cup. Boil for 2 or 3 seconds, infuse for 10 minutes. Sweeten if desired (preferably with honey). 3 to 4 cups a day, during or after meals.
- general use in cooking (soups, grills, etc; see also Note 2 below).
- *essential oil*: use either in drops (3 to 5 drops 3 times a day in an alcoholic solution or in honey water) or *pills*:

essence of thyme.................................
almond soap .... } 0.10g of each
marsh mallow powder...........................
4 to 6 pills daily, after meals.
- in conjunction with eucalyptus and cypress to treat *whooping cough*.
- for tonsillitis, sore throat: chew thyme leaves.

N.B.
1. Infusion of thyme, which has a very pleasant flavour, cannot be recommended too highly as a substitute for tea or coffee at breakfast-time.
2. Recipe for a marinade, passed on by H. Leclerc:

> Steep a small bunch of thyme in $\frac{1}{2}$ a litre of white wine, together with a small bunch of savory, a few shallots, 3 or 4 cloves of garlic, 2 bayleaves and a few cloves. Add 250g of salt, 15g of fresh ground pepper (C. Husson).

External use:
- in ointments (for dermatosis, counter-irritant in cases of rheumatism and muscular pain, chest rubs for whooping cough), lotions and creams in cosmetics, toilet waters (effective bactericide: Novi);
- often used in conjunction with lemon and bergamot;
- in soapy solutions to disinfect the hands (in surgery);
- in decoction in olive oil, in compresses for *sores*, *wounds*.
- *insect bites* and snake bites: the essence or crushed plant (first-aid
· treatment).
- to treat rheumatic pains, chopped thyme heated in a pan, placed on a gauze dressing and applied hot
- *aromatic bath:*
  500g of thyme boiled in 4 litres of water and added to the bath water (arthritis, gout, rheumatism, debility; in addition, this will aid expectoration by fluidifying mucus).
- alternatively, a useful formula given by H. Leclerc:

  essence of thyme.................................. 2g
  essence of origanum............................. 0.5g
  essence of rosemary 1g
  essence of lavender.............................. 1g
  sub-carbonate of soda 350g

  Quantity sufficient for a deep bath: fortifying, beneficial to arthritics.
- *mixture for inhaling:*

  menthol.. 0.25g
  balsam of Peru 5g
  essence of thyme............................... 10g
  90° alcohol...................................... 80g

  1 teaspoon to a bowl of very hot water. 2 to 3 inhalations a day. (See under *Pine* for another formula, and under *Eucalyptus* for a formula for inhalation tablets).

- concentrated decoction: a handful of thyme to a litre of water. Boil until reduced by half (*hair tonic*, preventing or halting hair loss).
- against *lice* and *scabies*: see under *Cinnamon*.
- see under *Origanum* for the formula for an ointment.
- see under *Cinnamon* for the formula for the liqueur "Parfait amour".

N.B.

Thyme is one of the aromatic herbs most used in medicine since the most ancient times (by doctors in Egypt, Etruria, Greece and Rome – Dioscorides, for instance, Hippocrates, Pliny and Virgil). Depending on the species, it contains from 0.10 to 1.5% essential oil. Its 2 phenols, thymol (see below) and carvacrol can be used in the same way as essence of thyme and are frequently included in pharmaceutical preparations.

Chamberland (the elder), demonstrated in 1887 the bactericidal action of the essence (notably in respect of the anthrax bacillus). Cadéac and Meunier studied its effect on the typhus and glanders bacilli in 1889, using microbic cultures in meatbroth; Morel and Rochaix in 1921–22 its effect on meningococcus, Eberth's bacillus, the diphtheria bacillus and staphylococcus; Courmont, Morel and Bay its effect on the tuberculosis bacillus. Miquel had shown the bactericidal power of vapours of thyme (essence) in 1894.

Essence of thyme is a much stronger antiseptic than phenol (Mayer and Gottlieb), peroxide of hydrogen, potassium permanganate and guaiacol. Its bactericidal and cicatrising effects are far more profound in the *peroxidised* and *deterpenated* essences than in the unrefined essence, but it is necessary to use a suitable solvent to neutralise their irritant effect.

Peroxidised essence of thyme, at 0.10%, in a dilute soapy solution, destroys microbial flora in the mouth within 3 minutes (thyme dentifrices). Dried thyme in powdered form is a good dentifrice and strengthens the gums. It may be used mixed with clay in equal parts.

Novi (Italy) has demonstrated the stimulant effect of the essences of thyme, lavender and bergamot (similarly with lemon and camomile) on the white corpuscles, by which a "curative leucocytosis" is activated, enabling the body to combat toxins and to resist infectious diseases.

The essences produced by different species of thyme have noticeable differences in their chemical composition. Some contain a greater proportion of thymol, others of carvacrol and others again of citral (analogous to the essence of verbena). Nevertheless their properties are closely related.

Ylang-ylang

Cananga odorata

Annonanceae

The trees are native to the Far East – Java, Sumatra, the Philippines; also Madagascar, Réunion and the Comoro Islands, the best-known varieties coming from the Philippines, Réunion and the Comoros.

The *essence* is obtained by steam distillation of the flowers.

Principal known constituents:
linalol (both free and esterified), safrol, eugenol, geraniol, pinene, sesquiterpenses, cadinene, benzoate of benzyl, combined acetic, benzoic, formic, salicylic and valeric acids.

Properties:
- reduces hyperpnoea (over-accelerated breathing rate) and tachycardia (abnormal rapidity of heart-beat)
- *hypotensive*
- sedative (calming reflex excitability)
- *antiseptic*
- said to an aphrodisiac

Indications:
- *tachycardia*
- hypertension (high blood pressure)
- intestinal infections
- purulent secretions
- impotence, frigidity

Methods of use:
Internal:
- *essence*: 2 to 5 drops, three times a day, in an alcoholic solution or in honey water

External:
- the essence in aqueous emulsions or alcoholic solutions.

N.B.
Ylang-ylang is widely used in perfumery under several classifications according to its quality.

Before embarking on the Therapeutic Index, may I remind the reader that, like any form of treatment, Aromatherapy does not claim to be effective, by itself, for *every* ailment, nor for *every* patient, nor in *every* circumstance. It must often be used in conjunction with other medications.

---

3. Therapeutic Index of Ailments and the Aromatic Essences used in their Treatment.

Medical books are most often read by the layman, and to such a reader, who has a right to knowledge, I have also tried to be helpful. But it must be borne in mind that this section does not pretend to provide an exhaustive list of treatments; it presents no more than certain aspects of treatment which, according to the case, may be of great practical value or merely passing interest.

This book was in no way designed to take the place of diagnosis or the advice of a qualified practitioner. It must be emphasised that in any doubtful cause *a doctor must be consulted*. There is nothing more misleading than a "stomach-ache" which appears hardly worth bothering about. Two days later it may turn out to be peritonitis which neither doctor nor medicine can stop. Problems affecting eyesight are common, undoubtedly more common than the brain tumour of which they could be a symptom. . . . Medicine is full of snares – which is, I suppose, why medical training is so long; so long indeed that it never ends.

Moreover, diabetes, a gastric ulcer, colitis and any number of other diseases cannot be properly treated without clear guide-lines.

Nevertheless, the following pages may be found to be of service in numerous cases. They were, after all, written with that intention.

To make best use of this index, the reader should refer to the section in the preceding chapter dealing specifically with each essence mentioned here. There he will find the various methods of use, together with formulae, both ancient and modern, chosen for their proven worth.

ABRASIONS, see WOUNDS

ABSCESS, HOT: onion

ABSCESS, COLD: garlic

ACNE: cajuput, juniper, lavender

ADENITIS, ACUTE or CHRONIC: garlic, *onion*, pine, rosemary, sage

AEROPHAGY (swallowing of air): *aniseed, caraway, coriander,* fennel, *lemon, marjoram,* origanum, peppermint, tarragon

AGEING, see SENESCENCE

ALBUMINURIA: juniper

ALOPECIA: lavender, sage, thyme

AMENORRHOEA, see under MENSTRUATION

AMNESIA, see MEMORY, LOSS OF

ANAEMIA: camomile, garlic, lemon, thyme (infantile)

ANAL FISTULA: lavender, niaouli

ANGINA PECTORIS, FALSE (PSEUDO-ANGINA): aniseed, caraway, orange blossom

ANKYLOSTOMA DUODENALE, see HOOKWORM

ANOREXIA, see APPETITE, LOSS OF

ANTISEPTICS, Borneo camphor, cinnamon, eucalyptus, garlic, juniper, lavender, niaouli, pine, rosemary, thyme, ylang-ylang

ANTS, TO REPEL, see INSECTS, TO REPEL

ANXIETY: basil, lavender, marjoram, thyme

APHONIA, see VOICE, LOSS OF

APHTHAE, see THRUSH

APOPLEXY: sage

APPETITE, LOSS OF: bergamot *camomile*, caraway, coriander, fennel, garlic, ginger, hyssop, juniper, lemon, nutmeg, origanum, sage, tarragon

ARTERIOSCLEROSIS: *garlic*, juniper, *lemon*, *onion*

ARTERITIS (ARTERITIC SYNDROMES): garlic, lemon, marjoram, onion

ARTHRITIS: garlic, juniper, lemon, onion, thyme

ARTHROSIS, see RHEUMATISM, CHRONIC

ASCARIS, see ROUNDWORM

ASCITES: lemon, *onion*

ASTHMA: aniseed, cajuput, eucalyptus, *garlic*, *hyssop*, *lavender*, lemon, marjoram, niaouli, onion, origanum, peppermint, *pine*, *rosemary*, sage, savory, thyme

ATHEROSCLEROSIS, see ARTERIOSCLEROSIS

ATONY, GASTRIC: cinnamon, lavender, lemongrass, *origanum*, *sage*, *savory* (see also DYSPEPSIA, ATONIC)

AURAL NEURALGIA, see EARACHE

AZOTAEMIA (EXCESS UREA IN THE BLOOD): onion

BAD BREATH (DUE TO DYSPEPSIA): nutmeg, peppermint, rosemary, thyme

BALDNESS, see ALOPECIA

BED-WETTING, see ENURESIS

BILIOUS ATTACK: peppermint

BITES, ANIMAL: lavender, sage

BLADDER, see URINARY INFECTIONS

BLEPHARITIS, see EYELIDS, INFLAMMATION OF

BOILS: camomile, lemon, onion, thyme

BREAST-FEEDING PROBLEMS, see LACTATION

BREASTS, CONGESTION OF: fennel, geranium

BREATHLESSNESS, BREATHING DIFFICULTIES, see ASTHMA, PULMONARY DISEASES, RESPIRATORY DEFICIENCY

BRITTLENESS (NAILS): lemon

BRONCHITIC INFLUENZA: cinnamon, clove, eucalyptus, lemon, naiouli, thyme

BRONCHITIS, ACUTE: cajuput, *eucalyptus*, garlic, *lavender*, lemon, onion, *pine*, savory

BRONCHITIS, CHRONIC: cajuput, *'eucalyptus*, garlic, *hyssop*, lavender, lemon, *niaouli*, onion, *origanum*, peppermint, pine, rosemary, sage, sandalwood, savory, terebinth, thyme

BRUISES, see CONTUSIONS

BURNS: camomile, eucalyptus, geranium, *lavender*, niaouli, onion, rosemary, sage

CALCULUS, BILIARY or URINARY, see GALLSTONES or URINARY STONES

CALLOUSES: garlic

CALMATIVES: cinnamon, cypress, lavender (and aspic: cerebro-spinal excitation), marjoram, sage (antispasmodic), etc

CANCER, PREVENTION AND TREATMENT OF: clove, cypress, garlic, geranium, hyssop, onion, sage, tarragon

CANCER OF THE UTERUS: geranium, juniper (?)

CAPILLARY FRAGILITY: lemon

CARDIAC FATIGUE: aniseed, Borneo camphor, garlic

CARBUNCLE: see furunculosis

CARDIO-VASCULAR ERETHISM: aniseed, caraway

CATARRH, NASAL, see CORYZA

CATARACT: ginger (?)

CELLULITIS (PAINS): cypress, origanum

CEREBRAL CONGESTION: onion

CHANGE OF LIFE: see MENOPAUSE

CHAPPED SKIN: onion

CHILBLAINS: lemon, onion

CHILDBIRTH, PREPARATION FOR: *clove, sage*

CHILDREN, DEBILITY IN, see under DEBILITY

CHILL: cinnamon, thyme (see also INFLUENZA)

CHLORAEMIA: onion

CHLOROSIS (GREEN SICKNESS): lavender, pine, *rosemary*, thyme

CHOLECYSTITIS (INFLAMMATION OF THE GALL-BLADDER): pine, *rosemary*

CHOLERA: cinnamon, eucalyptus, peppermint, sage

CHOLESTEROL, EXCESS OF: rosemary, thyme

CICATRISING (HEALING) AGENTS: cajuput, camomile, clove, eucalyptus, garlic, *hyssop*, juniper, *lavender*, niaouli, onion, *rosemary*, *sage*, savory, terebinth, thyme

CIRCULATORY DISORDERS: cypress, garlic, lemon, thyme

CIRRHOSIS: juniper, *onion*, rosemary

COLDS, see BRONCHITIS, INFLUENZA

COLDS IN THE HEAD, see CORYZA

COLIBACILLOSIS: *eucalyptus*, *sandalwood*, etc

COLIC, see INTESTINAL COLIC

COLITIS, see INTESTINAL INFECTIONS

COLITIS, SPASMODIC, see SPASM, INTESTINAL
CONDYLOMA: thuja
CONGESTION OF THE LIVER, see HEPATIC CONGESTION
CONJUNCTIVITIS: camomile, lemon
CONSTIPATION: rosemary, terebinth
CONTAGIOUS DISEASES, PROPHYLAXIS and TREATMENT: cinnamon, clove, eucalyptus, garlic, ginger, juniper
CONTUSIONS: aromatic tincture of arnica (aniseed, *cinnamon*, clove, ginger); fennel, hyssop, sage
CONVALESCENCE: Borneo camphor, lemon, *sage*, thyme
CONVULSIONS: camomile
CORNS: garlic
CORYZA: basil (CHRONIC CORYZA), cinnamon, lemon, marjoram, niaouli, onion, peppermint, thyme (CATARRH)
COUGH: aniseed, *eucalyptus*, hyssop
COUGH, SPASMODIC or CONVULSIVE: *cypress*, eucalyptus, hyssop, lavender, origanum, *thyme*
COUGHING BLOOD, see HAEMOPTYSIS
CRAB-LICE, see LICE
CRACKED SKIN: onion
CUTS, see WOUNDS
CYSTS: garlic
CYSTITIS: cajuput, eucalyptus, fennel, juniper, lavender, niaouli, *pine*, sandalwood, terebinth, thuja, thyme
DEAFNESS: fennel, garlic, onion, savory
DEBILITY, GENERAL: basil, *Borneo camphor*, cinnamon, clove, eucalyptus, garlic, geranium, ginger, hyssop, lavender, lemon, marjoram, nutmeg, *onion*, *peppermint*, pine, *rosemary*, *sage*, *thyme* (see also MENTAL FATIGUE and NERVOUS DEBILITY)
DEBILITY, INFANTILE: lavender, marjoram, pine, rosemary, sage
DEBILITY, INFLUENZAL: *cinnamon*, lemon, sage, thyme
DECALCIFICATION: lemon
DEMINERALISATION: lemon
DENTALGIA, see TOOTHACHE
DEPRESSIVE STATES, see NERVOUS DEPRESSION
DERMATITIS, see DERMATOSIS
DERMATOSIS: cajuput, camomile, geranium, hyssop, juniper (cade oil), sage, thyme
DIABETES: eucalyptus, *geranium*, *juniper*, onion
DIARRHOEA: camomile, cinnamon, clove, garlic, geranium, ginger, juniper, *lavender*, lemon, nutmeg, onion, orange blossom (chronic), peppermint, rosemary, sage, sandalwood (persistent), *savory*
DIARRHOEA, INFANTILE: camomile, onion, sage
DIARRHOEA, IN TUBERCULAR PATIENTS: sage
DIGESTION, SLUGGISH OR PAINFUL, see ATONY, GASTRIC and DYSPEPSIA, ATONIC

DIPHTHERIA: garlic (prophylactic)
DISINFECTANT, DOMESTIC: eucalyptus, juniper, lavender, sage
DISTENSION OF THE STOMACH, see FLATULENCE
DIURETICS: cypress, juniper, *onion*, rosemary, sage, terebinth
DIZZINESS, see VERTIGO
DROPSY: garlic, juniper, *onion*, terebinth (see also OEDEMA)
DYSHIDROSIS: cypress, pine
DYSMENORRHOEA, see under MENSTRUATION
DYSPEPSIA: aniseed, basil, bergamot, *camomile*, cinnamon, clove, *coriander*, fennel, garlic, ginger, hyssop, juniper, lavender, lemon, lemongrass, onion, peppermint, sage, savory, *tarragon*, thyme
DYSPEPSIA, ATONIC: bergamot, *cinnamon*, *fennel*, garlic, ginger, hyssop, juniper, lavender, lemongrass, nutmeg, onion, *origanum*, *peppermint*, *rosemary*, *sage*, thyme
DYSPEPSIA, NERVOUS: aniseed, *caraway*, coriander, orange blossom, savory, tarragon
DYSPNOEA, see RESPIRATORY DEFICIENCY
EAR, INFLAMMATION OF: lemon, niaouli
EARACHE: cajuput, garlic
EARS, BUZZING IN: onion
ECCHYMOSIS, see CONTUSIONS
ECZEMA: camomile, hyssop, sage
ECZEMA, WEEPING: juniper
ECZEMA, DRY: geranium, lavender
EMMENAGOGUES: basil, camomile, caraway, cinnamon, fennel, hyssop, juniper, lavender, lavender cotton, nutmeg, origanum, peppermint, *rosemary*, *sage*, tarragon, *thyme*, (see MENSTRUATION)
ENDOCRINE GLANDS, see GLANDULAR IMBALANCE
ENTERITIS, see INTESTINAL INFECTIONS
ENURESIS: *cypress*, (thuja)
EPIDEMICS, PREVENTIVE OF: eucalyptus, garlic, juniper, lemon, niaouli
EPILEPSY: basil, cajuput, *rosemary*, terebinth, thyme
EXHAUSTION, see DEBILITY and MENTAL FATIGUE
EXOPHTHALMIC GOITRE: garlic, onion
EYELIDS, INFLAMMATION OF: camomile, lemon
FACE, CARE OF: lemon
FACIAL NEURALGIA: camomile, geranium
FAINTING: cinnamon, rosemary
FATIGUE, see DEBILITY and MENTAL FATIGUE
FATIGUE OF THE LIMBS: rosemary
FEBRILE STIFFNESS: cinnamon, *thyme*
FEET, IRRITATION OF: lemon
FEET, OFFENSIVELY SMELLING, see SWEATING, OFFENSIVE
FEVERISH STATES: eucalyptus, lemon, sage
FEVERS, ERUPTIVE: eucalyptus, hyssop, lavender

FLATULENCE: aniseed, basil, bergamot, camomile, caraway, cinnamon, clove, *coriander*, *fennel*, garlic, ginger, hyssop, lavender, lemon, marjoram, nutmeg, *onion*, origanum, *peppermint*, rosemary, sage, savory, *tarragon*, terebinth, thyme

FLEAS: essence of turpentine

FRECKLES: lemon, onion

FRIGIDITY, see IMPOTENCE

FURUNCLES, see BOILS

FURUNCULOSIS: thyme

GALLSTONES: *lemon*, nutmeg, *onion*, *pine*, rosemary, *essence of turpentine*

GASTRALGIA: cinnamon, *fennel*, geranium, hyssop, peppermint, pine, rosemary, savory, tarragon

GASTRITIS: lemon

GASTRITIS, CHRONIC, see APPETITE, LOSS OF and FLATULENCE

GASTRO-ENTERITIS: geranium (see also INTESTINAL INFECTIONS)

GASTRORRHAGIA (GASTRIC HAEMORRHAGE): lemon

GENITAL ERETHISM: marjoram

GENITO-URINARY INFECTIONS: juniper, lavender, niaouli, onion, thyme

GIDDINESS, see VERTIGO

GINGIVITIS: lemon, sage

GLANDULAR IMBALANCE: cypress, garlic, onion, sage

GLANDULAR INFLAMMATION, see ADENITIS

GLOSSITIS, see TONGUE, INFLAMMATION OF

GONORRHOEA: garlic, juniper, *lavender*, lemon, *sandalwood*

GOUT: basil, cajuput, camomile, fennel, *garlic*, *juniper*, lemon, pine, *rosemary*, terebinth, thyme

GROWING PAINS: lemon, onion

GUMS, CARE OF (TO STRENGTHEN): fennel, lemon, sage, thyme

HAEMOPHILIA: lemon, terebinth

HAEMOPTYSIS: cinnamon, cypress, geranium, juniper, lemon

HAEMORRHAGE, see GASTRORRHAGIA, HAEMOPTYSIS, INTESTINAL HAEMORRHAGE, NOSEBLEED, UTERINE HAEMORRHAGE

HAEMORRHOIDS: *cypress*, garlic, onion

HAIR, CARE OF: thyme

HAIR, LOSS OF: see ALOPECIA

HALITOSIS, see BAD BREATH

HANDS, CARE OF: lemon

HAY FEVER: hyssop

HEADACHE: *camomile* (influenzal), lavender, lemon, peppermint

HEART CONDITIONS OF NERVOUS·ORIGIN: rosemary (see also CARDIAC FATIGUE, PALPITATIONS)

HEPATIC CONGESTION: camomile, *lemon*, rosemary, thyme
HEPATIC DEFICIENCY: *lemon*
HEPATIC DISORDERS: lemon, peppermint, *rosemary*, sage, thyme
HERPES: geranium, lemon
HICCOUGH: tarragon
HIGH BLOOD PRESSURE, see HYPERTENSION
HOARSENESS, see VOICE, LOSS OF
HOOKWORM (ANKYLOSTOMA DUODENALE): thyme
HYPERCOAGULABILITY OF THE BLOOD: garlic lemon
HYPERTENSION (ARTERIAL): *garlic*, lavender, lemon, marjoram, ylang-ylang
HYPERVISCOSITY OF THE BLOOD: lemon
HYPOTENSION: hyssop, rosemary, *sage*, thyme
HYSTERIA: cajuput, camomile, lavender, rosemary
IMPETIGO: see DERMATOSIS
IMPOTENCE: aniseed (?), cinnamon, clover, ginger, juniper, *onion*, peppermint, *pine*, rosemary, sandalwood, *savory*, thyme, ylang-ylang
INDIGESTION, see DYSPEPSIA
INFECTIONS, VARIOUS: *Borneo camphor*, eucalyptus, garlic, lemon, onion, *pine*, . . . in fact all the essences are bactericidal
INFECTIOUS DISEASES, PROPHYLAXIS and TREATMENT: *Borneo camphor*, clove, eucalyptus, *garlic*, lavender, lemon, onion *pine*, *thyme* (see also CONTAGIOUS DISEASES)
INFLUENZA: Borneo camphor, camomile, *cinnamon* (post-influenzal debility), *cypress*, *eucalyptus*, fennel (prophylactic), *garlic*, (prophylactic), hyssop, *lavender*, *lemon*, niaouli, onion, peppermint, pine, rosemary, sage, *thyme*
INSECT BITES AND STINGS: basil, cinnamon, garlic, *lavender*, lemon, onion, sage, savory, thyme
INSECTS, TO REPEL: lemon (ANTS); clove, lavender, lemon (CLOTHES MOTHS); *eucalyptus*, clove, geranium, onion, peppermint (MOSQUITOS, GNATS, etc)
INTERCOSTAL NEURALGIA: peppermint
INTESTINAL COLIC: *aniseed* (infantile), *bergamot*, hyssop, peppermint
INTESTINAL HAEMORRHAGE: terebinth
INTESTINAL INFECTIONS, ENTERITIS, COLITIS: basil, bergamot, cajuput, camomile, cinnamon, *garlic*, geranium, hyssop, *lavender*, *lemongrass*, niaouli, rosemary, terebinth, *thyme*, ylang-ylang
INTESTINAL PAIN, see under SPASM
INTESTINAL PARASITES: *bergamot*, cajuput, camomile, caraway, cinnamon, clove, eucalyptus, fennel, garlic, hyssop, lavender, *lavender cotton*, lemon, niaouli, *onion*, peppermint, savory, terebinth (tapeworm), thuja, *thyme* (see also under ANGUILLULA, HOOKWORM, OXYURIS, ROUNDWORM, TAPEWORM, TRICHOCEPHALUS)
IRRITABILITY: camomile, cypress, lavender, marjoram

ITCHING: vinegar (Chapter 6)

JAUNDICE: geranium, lemon, rosemary, thyme

KIDNEYS, see URINARY INFECTIONS, etc, also STIMULANT, RENAL

LACTATION, TO STIMULATE: aniseed, caraway, fennel, lemongrass

LACTATION, TO DRY UP: peppermint, sage

LARYNGITIS: niaouli, onion

LARYNGITIS, CHRONIC: cajuput, sage

LEUCOMA CORNEAL: clove (?)

LEUCORRHOEA: cinnamon, *hyssop*, juniper, *lavender*, rosemary, sage, terebinth, thyme

LICE: cinnamon, eucalyptus, clove, geranium, lavender, lemon, lemongrass, mustard, origanum, rosemary, terebinth, thyme

LIMBS, see FATIGUE OF

LITHIASIS, BILIARY or URINARY, see GALLSTONES or URINARY STONES

LIVER, see under HEPATIC

LOSS OF APPETITE, see APPETITE, LOSS OF

LOSS OF HAIR, see ALOPECIA

LOSS OF MEMORY, see MEMORY, LOSS OF

LOSS OF VOICE, see VOICE, LOSS OF

LOW BLOOD PRESSURE, see HYPOTENSION

LUMBAGO, LUMBAR PAINS: camomile (resulting from influenza), geranium (see also RHEUMATIC PAINS)

LUNGS, see under PULMONARY DISEASES

LUPUS: clove

LYMPHATISM: lavender, *onion*, rosemary, sage

MALARIA: eucalyptus, lemon

MANGE: caraway, juniper

MEASLES: eucalyptus (prophylactic)

MELANCHOLIA, see NERVOUS DEPRESSION

MEMORY, LOSS OF: basil, clove, (coriander), *rosemary*

MENOPAUSE: camomile, *cypress*, *sage*

MENSTRUATION, ABSENCE OF (AMENORRHOEA): camomile, cypress, *origanum*, peppermint, sage, *thyme*

MENSTRUATION, DIFFICULT: caraway, juniper, lavender-cotton

MENSTRUATION, PAINFUL (DYSMENORRHOEA): aniseed, cajuput, camomile, *cypress*, juniper, *peppermint*, rosemary, *sage*, tarragon

MENSTRUATION, SCANTY, IRREGULAR: basil, cinnamon, *fennel*, lavender, lavender-cotton, nutmeg, peppermint, *sage*

MENTAL INSTABILITY: marjoram, thyme

MENTAL FATIGUE, MENTAL STRAIN: basil, clove, onion, *rosemary*, savory, thyme

METEORISM, see FLATULENCE

METRITIS, see LEUCORRHOEA

METRORRHAGIA, see UTERINE HAEMORRHAGE

MIGRAINE: aniseed, basil, *camomile*, *eucalyptus*, *lavender*, lemon, *marjoram*, onion, *peppermint*, *rosemary*, terebinth

MILK, see LACTATION

MOSQUITOS, TO REPEL, see INSECTS, TO REPEL

MOTHS, TO REPEL, see INSECTS, TO REPEL

MOUTH, INFLAMMATION OF (STOMATITIS): geranium, lemon, *sage*

MUSCULAR PAINS, see RHEUMATISM, MUSCULAR

MUSCULAR STIFFNESS: rosemary, thyme

NERVOUS CRISIS: camomile, lavender, thyme

NERVOUS DEBILITY (NEURASTHENIA): *basil*, coriander, lavender, marjoram, *sage*, thyme

NERVOUS DEPRESSION: *Borneo camphor*, *camomile*, lavender, thyme

NERVOUS STATES: lavender, marjoram, *orange blossom*, verbena

NERVOUS SYSTEM, TO BALANCE: aspic (lavender), *cypress*, lavender, rosemary, sage

NETTLE-RASH (URTICARIA): camomile

NEURALGIA, see under FACIAL, INTERCOSTAL and RHEUMATIC

NOSEBLEED: lemon, terebinth

OBESITY: lemon, onion

OEDEMA: garlic, geranium, *onion* (see also DROPSY)

OLIGURIA: aniseed, *fennel*, garlic, *juniper*, lavender, *onion*, sage, terebinth

OPHTHALMIA: camomile, geranium

ORAL HYGIENE: thyme

OTITIS, see EAR, INFLAMMATION OF

OVARIES, (ovarian problems): cypress, sage

OXYURIS (PIN-WORM, THREADWORM): camomile, *eucalyptus*, garlic, lavender-cotton, lemon, thyme

PALPITATIONS: *aniseed*, caraway, orange blossom, *peppermint*, rosemary

PALUDISM, see MALARIA

PANCREATIC DEFICIENCY: lemon

PAPILLOMA, see WARTS

PARALYSIS: basil, peppermint, sage

PARALYSIS, AFTER-EFFECTS OF: *juniper*, *lavender*, *rosemary*

PEDICULOSIS, see LICE

PELVIC CONGESTION: thuja

PERICARDITIS: onion

PERIODS, see MENSTRUATION

PHARYNGITIS, CHRONIC: cajuput

PHLEBITIS: lemon

PHOSPHORUS POISONING: terebinth

PILES, see HAEMORRHOIDS

PLETHORA, garlic, lemon
PLEURISY: onion
PNEUMONIA: eucalyptus, lavender, lemon, niaouli, pine
POISONING, GASTRO-INTESTINAL: peppermint (see also PHOSPHORUS POISONING, SNAKE BITES)
POLYP: thuja
POST-INFLUENZAL DEBILITY, see DEBILITY, INFLUENZAL
PREVENTION, PROPHYLAXIS: see CONTAGIOUS DISEASES, INFECTIOUS DISEASES
PROSTATE, ENLARGEMENT OF: onion, thuja
PROSTATITIS: *pine*
PRURITIS, see ITCHING
PRURITIS, VULVAR: camomile, thyme
PSORIASIS: cajuput
PUBERTY: garlic, cypress, onion, pine, thyme
PUERPERAL INFECTION: niaouli, terebinth
PULMONARY DISEASES: cajuput, clove, cypress, *eucalyptus*, fennel, *garlic*, hyssop, lavender, lemon, niaouli, onion, origanum, peppermint, pine, sage, sandalwood, terebinth, *thyme* (see also ASTHMA, BRONCHITIS, etc)
PULMONARY EMPHYSEMA: cypress, *garlic*, hyssop, *thyme*
PULMONARY GANGRENE: eucalyptus, garlic
PULMONARY HAEMORRHAGE, see HAEMOPTYSIS
PULMONARY MYCOSIS, thyme
PULMONARY TUBERCULOSIS: cajuput, clove, *eucalyptus*, *garlic*, hyssop, lavender, *lemon*, *niaouli*, *origanum*, peppermint, *pine*, sage, *terebinth*, thyme
PURIFICATION OF DRINKING WATER: lemon, niaouli
PUTREFACTIVE FERMENTATION: caraway, cinnamon, *clove*, juniper, onion, *savory*, *tarragon*, thyme
PYELITIS: pine, terebinth, thyme
PYORRHOEA ALVEOLARIS, see GINGIVITIS
RACHITIS, see RICKETS
RESPIRATORY DEFICIENCY: aniseed, cinnamon, garlic, hyssop
RESPIRATORY INFECTIONS, see PULMONARY DISEASES
RHEUMATIC PAINS (RHEUMATIC NEURALGIA): cajuput, camomile, coriander, eucalyptus, garlic, ginger, lavender, marjoram, nutmeg, origanum, tarragon, terebinth
RHEUMATISM, CHRONIC: cajuput, camomile, cypress, *eucalyptus*, *garlic*, hyssop, *juniper*, lavender, *lemon*, niaouli, onion, *origanum*, pine, rosemary, tarragon, *terebinth*, *thyme*
RHEUMATISM, MUSCULAR: origanum, rosemary, thyme
RHINITIS: basil, *niaouli*, *thyme*
RICKETS: onion, pine, sage, thyme
ROUNDWORM (ASCARIS): camomile, *eucalyptus*, garlic, lavender-cotton, *thyme*

SCABIES: caraway, cinnamon, clove, garlic, lavender, lemon, mustard, peppermint, pine, rosemary, terebinth, thyme

SCALP, see ALOPECIA and HAIR

SCARLET FEVER: eucalyptus (prophylactic)

SCIATICA: terebinth

SCROFULOSIS: lavender, onion, sage

SCURF, camomile, geranium, lemon

SCURVY: ginger, *lemon*, *onion*

SEDATIVES: camomile, lavender, lemon, marjoram, thyme (see also CALMATIVES)

SENESCENCE: garlic, lemon, onion, thyme

SHINGLES: geranium; citral, magnesium and *tegarome*

SIGHT, POOR or WEAK: rosemary

SINUSITIS: eucalyptus, lavender, lemon, niaouli, peppermint, pine, thyme

SKIN, CHAPPED: onion

SKIN, CRACKED: onion

SKIN, GREASY, see FACE, CARE OF

(see also DERMATOSIS, ECZEMA, etc)

SNAKE BITES: anti-venom serum with basil, cinnamon, lavender, lemon or thyme as supplementary or first-aid treatment

SORES, see WOUNDS

SPASM: *coriander*, cypress, lavender, lavender-cotton, marjoram, terebinth

SPASM, CARDIAC: orange blossom

SPASM, DIGESTIVE, aniseed, *cinnamon*, *coriander*, marjoram

SPASM, GASTRIC: *basil*, cajuput, *caraway*, peppermint

SPASM, INTESTINAL: *aniseed*, *bergamot*, cajuput, *camomile*, caraway, cinnamon, clove, fennel, garlic, *lavender*, *peppermint*, pine, savory, *tarragon*, terebinth

SPASM, VASCULAR: cypress, garlic

SPASMODIC COUGH, see COUGH, SPASMODIC

SPERMATORRHOEA: lavender, marjoram

SPIDER BITES, see INSECT BITES AND STINGS

SPITTING BLOOD, see HAEMOPTYSIS

STIFFNESS: see under FEBRILE or MUSCULAR

STIMULANTS OF ADRENAL CORTEX: Borneo camphor, geranium, pine, rosemary, sage, savory

STIMULANTS, BULBAR: hyssop

STIMULANTS, CARDIAC: rosemary

STIMULANTS, CIRCULATORY and RESPIRATORY: cinnamon

STIMULANTS, OF NERVOUS SYSTEM: basil, rosemary, sage, savory

STOMACH AND INTESTINAL CRAMPS IN CHILDREN: camomile

STOMACH PAINS, see GASTRALGIA

STOMATITIS, see MOUTH, INFLAMMATION OF

SUCKLING, see LACTATION
SWEATING, OFFENSIVE (OF FEET AND ARMPITS): cypress, pine
SWEATING, PROFUSE: *sage* (IN TUBERCULAR PATIENTS AND CONVALESCENTS), thyme
SYMPATHETIC NERVOUS SYSTEM, DYSTONIA OF: lemongrass, origanum, rosemary, tarragon
SYPHILIS: lemon
SYPHILITIC SORES, CHANCRES: lavender
TACHYCARDIA: garlic, *ylang-ylang*
TAENIA, see TAPEWORM
TAPEWORM: garlic, *terebinth*, thyme
TEETH, CARE OF: aniseed, *clove*, lemon, peppermint, thyme
TEETHING: camomile
THREADWORM, see OXYURIS
THROAT, SORE: geranium, ginger, lemon, sage, thyme
THRUSH (APHTHAE): geranium, lemon, *sage*
TICS: marjoram (see also FACIAL NEURALGIA)
TINEA: garlic, lemon
TONSILLITIS: geranium, ginger, lemon, sage, thyme
TOOTHACHE: cajuput, cinnamon, clove, garlic, juniper, (Cade oil), nutmeg, onion, peppermint, sage
TRACHEITIS: pine
TREMORS: peppermint, rosemary, sage
TUBERCULOSIS, PULMONARY, see PULMONARY TUBER-CULOSIS
TYPHOID FEVER: cinnamon, garlic, lavender, lemon, thyme
TYPHUS: eucalyptus
ULCERS, STOMACH (GASTRIC) and INTESTINAL (DUODENAL): *camomile, geranium,* lemon
ULCERS, LEG (VARICOSE), see WOUNDS, ATONIC
UREA IN THE BLOOD, EXCESS, see AZOTAEMIA
URETHRITIS: cajuput, niaouli, terebinth
URIC ACID, EXCESS: lemon
URINARY INFECTIONS, DISORDERS OF THE URINARY TRACT: cajuput, eucalyptus, fennel, geranium, *juniper*, lavender, lemon, niaouli, onion, pine, sage, sandalwood, terebinth, *thyme*
URINARY STONES: *fennel, garlic, geranium, hyssop, juniper, lemon*
URINE, SCANT, see OLIGURIA
URTICARIA, see NETTLE-RASH
UTERINE HAEMORRHAGE (METRORRHAGIA): cinnamon, *cypress*, geranium, juniper, terebinth
VARICOSE VEINS: *cypress*, garlic, lemon
VEGETATIONS (plant-like growths): hyssop, thuja
VENEREAL DISEASES, see GENITO-URINARY INFECTIONS, GONORRHOEA, SYPHILIS
VERRUCA: *garlic*, lemon, onion, *thuja*

VERTIGO: *aniseed*, basil, camomile, caraway, *lavender*, peppermint, *rosemary*, sage, thyme
VOICE, LOSS OF: cypress, lemon, thyme
VOMITING: lemon, peppermint
VOMITING, NERVOUS: aniseed, cajuput, fennel, peppermint
WARTS: *garlic*, lemon, onion, *thuja*
WASP STINGS, see INSECT BITES AND STINGS
WEAKNESS, see DEBILITY
WHITLOW: onion
WHOOPING COUGH: *basil*, *cypress*, *garlic*, *lavender*, niaouli, origanum, rosemary, terebinth, thyme
WIND, see FLATULENCE
WORMS, see INTESTINAL PARASITES
WOUNDS, SORES, CUTS, etc: cajuput, *camomile*, clove, *eucalyptus*, garlic, geranium, hyssop, juniper, *lavender*, niaouli, onion, rosemary, sage, savory, thyme
WOUNDS, ATONIC (ULCERS, etc): cajuput, clove, garlic, juniper, lavender, niaouli, onion, rosemary, sage, savory, terebinth, thyme
WOUNDS, INFECTED: cajuput, camomile, clove, eucalyptus, garlic, lavender, onion, rosemary, savory, terebinth
WRINKLES: lemon

4. Some Formulae for Prescriptions in current use.

N.B.
E.O. = "essential oil"
q.s.f. = quantity sufficient for

This chapter sets out some simple formulae to be used in the treatment of various complaints which respond well to aromatherapy.

1. *For pulmonary complaints* (colds, influenza, bronchitis, tuberculosis, etc), to be used alone or in conjunction with other treatments, as a curative or a preventive:

E.O. thyme	⎫
E.O. niaouli....................................	⎬ 1g of each
E.O. pine needles	⎭
E.O. mint.......................................	0.50g
Alcohol at 90°	q.s.f. 60ml

25 drops in half a glass of lukewarm water, 10 minutes before meals, 3 times a day. *Dosage for children*, from 3 to 10 drops 3 times a day according to age.

*Friction rub for the chest:

Camphor	1g
Chloroform	5g
E.O. eucalyptus.................................	5g
E.O. pine	10g
Mustard	0.025g
Glycerine	20g
Alcohol at 90°	q.s.f. 90ml

rub on the chest morning and night (for children under 10 years I would recommend mustard plasters or applications of tincture and iodine).

2. *For intestinal complaints* (enteritis, colitis, parasitosis):

E.O. lavender	⎫
E.O. savory	⎬ 0.75g of each
E.O. basil.....................................	⎭
E.O. caraway...................................	
Alcohol at 90°	q.s.f. 60ml

213

25 to 40 drops in half a glass of lukewarm water, 10 minutes before meals, 3 times a day. For children, see the therapeutic index which refers back to the plants.

*Also effective: charcoal, bilberries, clay, oral vaccines, *pollen*: see also therapeutic index.

3. *For circulatory complaints:*

E.O. cypress....................................	1g
E.O. lavender	
E.O. sage	} 0.75g of each
E.O. thyme	
Alcohol at 90°............................ q.s.f. 60 ml	

Same dosage.

*It is worth remembering hydrastis, witch hazel and horse chestnut, which are contained in numerous proprietary medicines, in the treatment of such complaints.

4. *For infections of the urinary tract:*

E.O. cajuput	
E.O. lavender	
E.O. juniper....................................	} 0.75g of each
E.O. niaouli....................................	
Alcohol at 90°............................ q.s.f 60ml	

Same dosage

*Also effective: sandalwood, methylene blue, oral vaccines, magnesium.

5. *For rheumatic complaints:*

E.O. juniper....................................	1g
E.O. thyme	0.50g
E.O. cypress....................................	0.50g
E.O. sassafras..................................	1g
E.O. turpentine.................................	0.50g
Alcohol at 90°............................ q.s.f. 60ml	

Same dosage.

*For arthrosis, iodine and sulphur may also be used.

6. *For all rheumatic or muscular pains*, a mixture consisting of:

Tincture of ginger..............................	180g
E.O. origanum	6g
E.O. juniper....................................	6g
E.O. camomile	2g
E.O. turpentine.................................	15g
Spirit of rosemary......................... q.s.f. 500ml	

Rub the painful areas morning and night (or more often if necessary).

214

7. *Formula to be prescribed in cases of senescence, loss of memory, etc:*

      E.O. rosemary................................... 1g
      E.O. sage ....
      E.O. savory ....
      E.O. basil...................................... } 0.50g of each
      E.O. ginger....................................
      Alcohol at 90°............................ q.s.f. 60ml

25 drops in half a glass of lukewarm water, 10 minutes before meals, 3 times daily.

*In certain cases, the following may also be used: wheatgerm, phosphorus, magnesium, pollen and royal jelly.

8. *To treat cases of loss of concentration,* use the following prescription to supplement treatments with lecithin, phosphorus or magnesium:

      E.O. basil......................................
      E.O. savory ....
      E.O. thyme .... } 50g of each
      E.O. marjoram ....
      E.O. rosemary.................................
      Alcohol at 90°............................ q.s.f. 60ml

10 drops in a little lukewarm water, 2 or 3 times a day before meals.

N.B.

As I have mentioned earlier in this book and think it worth repeating here, these preparations can only be made with *pure, natural essences* (an unfashionable concept, alas, in an era characterised by the synthetic) and these essences *in their complete form*. It is no use replacing essence of eucalyptus with eucalyptol (one of its constituents), for instance, nor essence of mint with menthol, etc.

5. Some Case Histories

This chapter sets out a few case histories of diseases treated with plants and aromatic essences in association with biological treatments.

It should of course be understood that not all results are as impressive as these – a fact I have emphasised and repeated throughout this and other works. But that such results are possible in some of the most severe and distressing cases is surely worth serious consideration.

The first case is that of a woman of 25 who had suffered from *recurring cystitis* since 1953. Urine tests continually showed the presence of the colon bacillus, staphylococcus and blood in quite considerable quantity. The disease had resisted all forms of treatment over a period of 7 years, that is until June 1960.

The woman was 1m 69cm (5ft 6in) tall and weighed only 48kg (7½ stone). Her general state of health was poor, and she suffered from extreme fatigue together with an exacerbated nervous condition. Lack of appetite, migraines, nausea, constipation and complaints linked to a malfunctioning sympathetic nervous system (palpitations, insomnia, etc) characterised the condition she was used to. The treatment recommended to her consisted of aromatic essences, plants given in the form of tinctures and a syrup of phosphoric acid base. She was also treated for poor circulation with infusions of a mixture of specially prepared plants, and put on a special diet.

In August 1960, two months after the start of this treatment, the patient told me that *the symptoms of cystitis had disappeared the day after the treatment had begun;* most of the other symptoms had also vanished and the only remaining problems were a mild sensation of fatigue and some palpitations.

In January 1961, after a treatment consisting exclusively of phyto-therapy and aromatherapy carried out at intervals, her general state of health was excellent; the cystitis, in particular, had not recurred.

Another case history, concerning a woman of 57 who came to consult me in July 1959, involved some *very severe symptoms indeed. For several years*, this woman had suffered from *daily attacks of vomiting* accompanied by extremely painful heartburn, as well as frequent pains caused by calculi in the gall-bladder and severe pains due to multiple arthrosis. Her general state of health was deplorable and – as might be

217

expected – tests showed *disturbing imbalances* in her blood count, sedimentation rate and calcium and phosphorus levels in the blood, etc. X-rays taken in the stomach region revealed a hiatus hernia with considerable oesophageal reflux.

The sick woman had undergone numerous operations over a period of 17 years – in particular several on the Fallopian tubes, another necessitated by peritonitis, and the removal of the thyroid. She had then refused to undergo any further surgery.

She was prescribed a treatment consisting entirely of aromatic essences and plants, in the form of powders, tinctures or decoctions: sap of wild lime, powder of horsetail, raphanus (horse-radish). An additional treatment of 1 teaspoon of powdered clay in half a glass of water first thing each morning was prescribed, to counteract most effectively the gastric and oesophageal pains which had made her existence particularly wretched, Some modifications to the diet were also recommended.

After 10 days of this treatment: the vomiting and heartburn had disappeared and her general state of health showed a marked improvement. Two months later, the symptoms were reduced by half.

After a further two months the patient had recovered, in her own words, "her old vitality". The vomiting attacks had never recurred, she was no longer in pain, and she had gained 3kg (more than 6lbs) in weight.

Eight months afterwards, tests showed that she had indeed made a complete recovery.

In September 1963, more than four years after the start of the treatment, the results were maintained in every respect with the aid of occasional phytotherapy and aromatherapy.

In 1968 the patient was still free from any recurrence of her former illnesses.

The third case concerns a 10-year-old child who underwent surgery for gangrenous appendicitis in 1953. Three days after the operation complications set in very quickly with a high fever (39°C) accompanied by enlargement of the lower abdomen. Forty-eight hours later, an incision was made to drain a gangrenous abscess from the right iliac fossa. The boy then began vomiting bile, suffering at the same time a total stoppage of solids and gas. Despite intensive care, the vomiting persisted and became blackish in colour. He was treated with penicillin and other antibiotics together with liver extracts, but developed pleurisy of the right lung on the 17th day, producing a fetid pus that contained "abundant and varied microbic flora". The child's condition was causing considerable concern and transfusions were considered necessary.

Three days later, in the face of this extremely grave situation, treatment based on aromatic essences and plants was begun, administered both orally and via the rectum. Two days later, it proved necessary to make a second incision to drain another accumulation of pus in the lower abdomen.

218

Two supplementary transfusions were then given and a few days later the child's general condition had improved. This was followed by a *normal recovery and convalescence.*

The treatment with aromatic essences had been administered over a total period of only six weeks (Dr G at St-P, Allier).

Eight years later, the child, by then a young man of 19, was still in excellent health.

I published in 1959, in the periodical "L'Hôpital"[1], some of the results which aromatherapy had been able to achieve in certain cases of *urinary and biliary lithiasis* (urinary and gall stones). Here are two examples:

, *The first* concerns a woman of 38 who had suffered gall-bladder attacks for several months. Frequent vomiting of bile and loss of appetite had caused her to lose 8kg (over a stone) in weight in six months, accompanied by extreme fatigue, an ashen complexion and severe constipation. An X-ray revealed the presence of a number of stones in her gall-bladder.

An aromatic treatment was prescribed for her, and after six weeks this brought about the expulsion of the gallstones. The process of elimination, causing little discomfort, lasted about an hour.

The patient put on 5kg (11lbs) in weight during the next two months and regained her strength and health. Six months later, X-rays showed that her gall-bladder was normal once again. Six years later, she was free from any recurrence, and was still in excellent health.

The second case is that of a woman of 44, who also suffered considerable pain from gallstones. A sudden and very painful attack indicated the need for immediate treatment. The patient's preference was for a treatment based on essences, which she began the following day.

Some days later, she eliminated 5 stones about the size of hazelnuts and, during the next few days, a blackish gravel containing a sixth stone, cylindrical in shape. Two days later, a clinical examination proved painless.

There were no further attacks during the next few years. The patient had recovered perfect health.

It must always be understood that where these complaints are concerned, 100% positive results cannot always be obtained. It can happen that plants or aromatic essences are unable to bring about the elimination of these stones. Generally speaking, however, patients suffer no further pain from gall-bladder or kidneys. They regain their appetites and are often able to dispense altogether with special diets. These improvements constitute a transformation of their lives and, furthermore, blood tests show that their general state of health is also markedly improved.

In such cases the treatment has only succeeded in eliminating the sediment or sand, generally quite substantial in quantity. This allows the gall bladder to function efficiently once more and to tolerate the presence of the stones, which in turn is beneficial to the whole organism.

1 "Lithiases and aromatherapy" *(L'Hôpital* – May 1959).

There are, however, cases where natural treatments have no noticeable effect on the patient's condition, where it is necessary to resort to surgery. In these cases, inflamed lesions are generally found in the region of the gall bladder or neighbouring organs, and it is then obvious that it would have been impossible to bring about expulsion of the stones, since the gall bladder itself had ceased to function. The organ having become virtually a foreign body, serving no useful purpose and often causing discomfort or pain, it is usually necessary to remove it at the same time as the stones.

* * *

"It is one's duty, and therefore one's right, to perform an experiment on a patient at any time when it might save his life." (Claude Bernard)

"If we take into account the infinite variety of individual human beings, every act of therapy is a form of research and experimentation." (Georges Duhamel)

If plants and aromatic essences can produce results that often cannot be bettered in the treatment of numerous illnesses, it seems reasonable that, in order to give the best chance possible to seriously ill patients, we should use a combination of all treatments, preferably natural or biological ones, that have proved effective against a particular complaint. The one proviso is that the different treatments should "pull" in the same direction, as horses pull a coach.

Among these treatments we should include, in varying combinations according to each case, the following: sea-water, trace elements, clay, numerous minerals and metalloids, oral or injectable vaccines, wheatgerm, yeasts, pollen and packed cell therapy.

The primary importance of diet must also be remembered since we improve or impair our health several times a day depending on what we eat. Hippocrates said: "Some illnesses can only be treated by eating correctly". We should also recall the words of Jean Rostand, who said "every menu is a prescription".

In the preceding pages we have seen the many exceptional properties of plants and aromatic essences. But these medications have an additional property of supreme importance: that of increasing the efficacy of other forms of treatment, by eliminating waste and toxins from the tissues.

Like many others, I have made a particular study of cancer for a number of reasons. First, because it is regarded as "an evil that spreads terror" and it is the duty of a doctor, like that of a soldier, to attack the enemy that appears to be the strongest; secondly, because I have been fortunate enough to witness some spectacular cures or improvements in certain cases of cancer. The patients had all been given only a short time to live by doctors who refuse to accept that medications that have not yet received official approval according to the tenets of our times can have any therapeutic value whatsoever. In *L'Officine* (1848), however, F. Dorvault wrote that "merely because their therapeutic properties have not yet received what one might call 'scientific consecration', it cannot be right to reject certain substances whose beneficial effects have been proved by practical experience."

For centuries it has been recognised that certain plants and essences are effective against tumours and cancers. I have attempted to reassess, these treatments in the light of present-day scientific knowledge.

In doing so, I have, in a number of cases where unexpected results were obtained, been able to confirm the truth of many of the beliefs on which ancient medicine is based.

I am also interested in the problem of cancer because many case histories have been published which involve *spontaneous* cures or remissions. I recall one case of gastric cancer which was discovered by surgery and considered inoperable, but which disappeared some months later following another operation necessitated by a completely different cause. It is possible that we come near to producing similar results in other cases. This phenomenon seems to indicate that, whatever the complexity of the cancer, all cases should be treated as if the object of the therapy were a total cure.

If we proceed upon these lines, it sometimes does happen that the results are unexpected and inexplicable. For, contrary to what one might expect, cancer patients can die even when they might seem to have been treated at a very early stage and when, at the outset, their general state of health might have appeared satisfactory. On the other hand, gravely ill patients, sometimes bed-ridden, can on occasion be transformed in a matter of weeks, and several years later appear to be completely restored to health. "What we refuse to accept is that a doctor, even when his skills have been proved powerless, can stand by inactive and watch the ravages of this disease" - the words of Dorvault once again. "For" he adds, "*this would be tantamount to saying that there is nothing new to discover in the field of therapy*, that all research and experiments are useless." It is this negative attitude, so often encountered, that drives patients towards the ranks of faith healers, genuine or otherwise, and towards hypnotists, skilled or not – in short, towards all those who claim to make up for the deficiencies of qualified doctors.

But facts cannot be disputed. Some patients regarded as doomed finding themselves in excellent health several years later, it seemed to me necessary to record a number of case histories in order to show that there are always reasons for hope.

In all the following cases, *phytotherapy and aromatherapy were used as the basic treatment.*

221

Cancers – four case histories.

The first case relates to a young girl of 19 who was first seen in 1958 for a **sarcoma of the left arm**. The surgeon, a friend of the family, operated on the tumour which was the size of an orange. "It was necessary, he wrote "to detach the arteries and nerves which passed through it (the humeral artery and the median and cutaneous brachial nerves). Even then, some tumorous tissue remained attached to them. The tumour spread along the length of the biceps and up towards the scapula."

The prognosis was evidently very grave at that stage. The patient was given radiotherapy and cobalt treatment, but it was thought that she could not live more than a few months.

I saw the patient in May 1958, two months after her operation. The scar was healing perfectly and there was no sign of secondary growths. However, her general state of health was poor, accompanied by a noticeable loss of weight. She had difficulty straightening her arm and flexing her fingers and the third and fourth fingers had grown claw-shaped.

A treatment was prescribed for her based on aromatic essences, phosphoric acid and magnesium. The treatment also included natural intestinal antiseptics (as used in most chronic complaints), together with various injectable substances recommended in the treatment of cancer.

Although I am not a homoeopath, I decided, because of the gravity of her condition, to add to this a local treatment of vaxinum, toxinum, cuprum, thuja, linoleic acid and kalicarbonicum.

The treatment was of course complemented by a *healthy diet* free of toxins – raw fresh vegetables, unrefined sunflower oil, leavened bread, etc.

In September 1958, 4 months after the start of the treatment, the patient had regained her appetite and was in an excellent state of health. She had gained 3kg (6½lbs) in weight and had recovered her vitality. She had also recovered full use of her hand and arm and, to this day, has had no further trouble from that source.

The aromatic treatment was continued *without interruption* and she was given 15 initial sessions of negative ionisation,[2] with further sessions following.

Apart from the *aromatic-based treatment*, other treatments included trace elements, magnesium, various minerals and packed cell therapy.

In February 1959, ten months after the start of the treatment, the patient was suddenly taken ill, in my absence, with a spontaneous pneumothorax of the left side accompanied by pleural effusion. The results of blood tests were disturbing, particularly the sedimentation rate. Half a litre of cloudy liquid was drawn off by puncture of the lung, but the culture remained sterile.

---

2   This treatment was developed by Charles Laville. Its aim is to restore to the body the negative electric charge which it has lost. In certain complaints, especially cancer, the electro-positivity of the body is too great, and can be neutralised by this treatment.

A course of treatment was prescribed comprising aromatic essences combined with natural vitamins and a concentrated potion of calcium chloride.

Since the patient's general condition was very grave and since it did not seem that surgery would be beneficial in this case, it was decided, at the formal request of the family, not to operate as had originally been intended.

Three months later, her general condition was excellent once again, tests proved normal, and she had regained the weight previously lost. In addition, *X-rays showed that the effusion had completely disappeared.* The lung, completely retracted at the beginning, had regained its normal position.

Now in September 1975, the patient is enjoying remarkably good health. Tests performed once a year prove satisfactory. It is now *more than 18 years* since the patient underwent her operation, at which stage she had been given only a few months to live.

The second case of cancer concerns a young man of 22, suffering from **a sarcoma of the outer edge of the right foot**, which had been discovered in November 1957. Two biopsies,[3] performed on 21st and 24th April 1958, confirmed that the sarcoma was of the fibroblast type. In May 1958 amputation at the hip was recommended.

On 7th May 1958, the very day when the amputation was to have been carried out, a general examination showed that the patient's general condition was poor, with a weight of 57kg (9$\frac{1}{2}$ stone) for a height of 1m 83cm (6 feet), and a wax-like complexion. The biopsy scar on the outer edge of the foot was suppurating and very painful to the touch, forcing the patient to limp.

The following treatment was prescribed: aromatherapy, administered internally, phosphoric acid, magnesium, and liver extracts. This was complemented by 15 sessions of *negative ionisation* and a diet of natural foods.

Three months later his general condition was good; there was no change locally.

Further treatment was administered as described above, with a basis of aromatic essences. The patient was also given trace elements and a further 30 sessions of ionisation.

The results of tests performed since that time have been indicated in previous publications.

Suffice it to say that this patient has had no further treatment since 1961. All tests have proved normal. In 14 months of treatment, the patient gained 19kg (3 stone). He is still in perfect health and is running a large business. His treatment consisted of aromatic essences and plants, supplemented by intra-muscular citral, trypanosa, trace elements prescribed on a temporary basis and packed cell therapy.

3 Biopsy: an operation which involves the removal of a minute piece of organ or tumour in order to examine the tissue under a microscope.

In December 1973, **16 years** after the discovery of the lesion, the patient was in perfect health.

The third case of cancer concerns a man of 51 who was seen in July 1959 for **cancer of the rectum** which apparently dated back to April of that year. This patient was suffering from rectal bleeding and fairly severe abdominal pain. He passed at least a dozen stools a day.

A rectal injection of barium revealed a "supra-rectal obstacle" accompanied by a stenosis extending along 5cm (2 inches) of the central part of the rectum. Tests showed certain abnormalities in the blood proteins and blood count.

The treatment consisted of aromatic plants and essences, magnesium, phosphoric acid, substances to restore the balance of the intestinal flora and aromatic enemas. In addition, trace elements and negative ionisation were administered. This therapy, with minor variations, was continued for 18 months, until December 1960.

X-rays, taken on 3 separate occasions, showed no change. However, in July 1960 the patient began to suffer from persistent constipation and occasionally passed stools tinged with blood. In December 1960 the presence of an occlusive syndrome necessitated an operation. The surgeon was unable to avoid the necessity for an iliac anus.

A histological examination revealed an infiltrating and vegetative glandular epithelioma of the rectum, but "fragments of tissue taken from each extremity of the resection were *free of cancerous cells* and the ganglions showed *no signs of metastasis*".

It is clear that surgical intervention was beneficial in this case, since it prevented the spread of the cancer.

In November 1967, 8½ years after the disease became apparent, the patient was in excellent health. He had a very strenuous manual job, and men of 30 working alongside him had difficulty keeping up with him. Tests had proved satisfactory on all counts.

We must, however, recognise that in some respects cancer is still a mystery to us. As a result of hepatic metastases detected in 1968, the patient died in September 1970; but the fact that this was *11½ years after* the disease was first detected must be attributed to the beneficial effects of the treatment.

The fourth example which I should like to mention concerns a woman of 57 who, as a result of an occlusion in July 1961, was found to be suffering from **cancer of the large intestine**.

She had a tumour in the left colonic flexure which had spread to the tail of the pancreas, the tissue surrounding the kidney and to the posterior abdominal wall. Excision of the tumour was impossible, so an anastomosis between the transverse and sigmoid colon was performed. "Removal of the affected tissue would have been impossible, as it would have meant sacrificing the left colonic flexure, the tail of the pancreas

224

and the spleen, while still leaving cancerous tissue in the abdominal wall."

Clearly, therefore, we were confronted with a very grave illness that left little room for hope. It was not expected that the patient would live more than a few months.

As soon as she left hospital on 23rd August 1961 the patient was treated with the various forms of therapy mentioned previously (aromatic essences, plants, magnesium, intestinal disinfectants, etc). Tests revealed severe disturbances in the body's biological functions.

In July 1962, the patient, who was living a virtually normal life and who had, because of this, somewhat neglected her treatment, suffered a sudden deterioration in her general condition. It was thought that she could not live more than a few weeks.

She was therefore required to follow a stricter course of treatment, for the most part biological medications and, in particular, aromatic essences.

An artificial anus formed spontaneously. From that time, the patient, although still of course underweight, ate and slept perfectly well, reading one or two books a day and moving around her apartment quite freely. In June 1963, contrary to all expectations, her condition was, if anything, improving, since she was gaining weight. To that day, *she had suffered no pain*, except at the time of the formation of her artificial anus.

In September 1963, two years after her operation, the general opinion was that she still had at least 18 months to live. However, she died 6 months later.

The case histories above have already been published in other medical books and in the earlier editions of this book, but I should like to add two others. Some of my colleagues have criticised me for having given an undue amount of attention to these cases, but I am of the opinion that even if a remission is all that is achieved this attention has been worthwhile.

The case of Mrs V
This patient came to see me in 1957, when she was 66. She had a swelling in her left breast which she had first noticed a year or two previously. The tumour was the size of a small hen's egg and lumpy. There were no external signs of cancerous growths and no ganglions. Her general health was excellent.

The results of blood tests were very unsatisfactory, which was to be expected, but I was reluctant in a case of this type to remove the lesion. The patient herself was also vehemently opposed to this operation.

I prescribed a treatment of based on phyto- and aromatherapy, magnesium, horsetail (for its silica content), carzodelan, trace elements, and *negative ionisation*.

225

This treatment was continued with various modifications for a year.

The results of tests taken at this time were normal. Strangely enough, however, although the tests remained excellent and her general health perfect, the tumour grew in size and became ulcerated. In 1962, I recommended a simple excision rather than large-scale mutilation as practised by Halsted, but the patient was still against any form of surgery.

Treatment was continued as before, supplemented by aromatic dressings to promote healing and prevent tissue degeneration.

In 1967 *(ten years later)* her general health was still excellent and tests normal.

One night the tumour began to bleed profusely and the patient was hospitalised immediately, The surgeon telephoned me, and the next day I left for the clinic 400 kilometres away.

In agreement with me, the surgeon carried out the simple removal of the breast, with no ganglionic curage, and no radiotherapy or cobalt treatment to follow.

The patient was given a series of treatments, all based on phyto- and aromatherapy, catalysis, magnesium, etc, and *negative ionisation.*

In December 1972, *17 years after the discovery of the disease,* Mrs V was still in very good health with a remarkably good general condition and normal test results. At the age of 82, she was still going about her daily life quite normally.

Points worth noting:
- The technique described above is not always so effective; we have to accept that some patients die whatever treatment they are given. Where cancer is concerned it should be recognised that all tumours are different, some "hares", some "birds", some "tortoises".
- But what should one's response be to the peremptory advice of a "grand master" among specialists who told me in 1965 that the patient had been very badly cared for and that there was nothing more that could be done for her? It was his method of treatment that, in this particular case, brought on phlebitis. It was evident that the treatment had to be modified, and this was done by various doctors acting solely on my advice.

It would be foolish to belive that these successes are due to the genius of the doctor − I wish merely to demonstrate that so much can be achieved, even the impossible, if we only try.

The second case concerns Mr F, who, *twelve years previously,* had undergone surgery for cancer of the right kidney. The operation was performed by Prof. N in a large Paris hospital.

The surgeon opened up the patient and, when he saw the damage the disease had caused, sewed up the incision *without doing anything.* The prognosis was clearly very grave. The patient was then referred to me.

I gave him a course of treatment similar to that administered in the previous case.

In 1974 the patient was in good health and was coping well with a very demanding job.

All that can be said is that *there is always something more that can be done before condeming a patient to death.* This idea is gradually gaining acceptance among doctors. it should also be remembered that the patients who do manage to survive these crises are those who still have the strength to fight. For, as Professor Hartmann wrote: "We can only help patients to fight for themselves".

*   *   *

I do not wish to overburden this book with detail, and from now on I shall limit myself to two case histories for each complaint studied.

Tuberculosis
Case No. 1: Mr D, aged 31 years.
This patient suffered from **bilateral pulmonary tuberculosis**, which had been diagnosed in 1948. He had had several relapses. In March 1958, resection of the ribs was recommended. He was given aromatic and local treatments, which produced excellent results after only a few months. Twelve years later (September 1970) he was still in good health.

Summary of patient's illness:
- hereditary antecedents: father suffered from pulmonary tuberculosis.
- antecedents among relatives: brother died of tuberculosis.
- personal antecedents: in 1948, at the age of 19, he suffered haemoptysis, caused by a cavity in the apex of the left lung. This was followed by a pneumothorax. The patient then spent two years in a sanatorium.

Resumption of activity in 1951 with the continuance of the pneumothorax until 1954.

In 1956 and 1957: patient suffered two bouts of jaundice and lost 12kg (about 2 stone) in weight.

In August 1957: cavity formed in the apex of the right lung.

The patient was treated in various establishments with **PAS**, streptomycin and rimifon over a period of six months. He then suffered double pneumoperitonitis.

In March 1958, since treatment had proved ineffective, *a thoracoplasty was recommended, but the patient refused to undergo this operation.*

March 1958: general state of health poor, with a weight of 68kg (10½ stone) for a height of 1m 83cm (6 feet). He suffered from severe disorders of the liver and digestive system – nausea, frequent vomiting and indigestion.

Treatment: aromatherapy, phosphoric acid, daily aromatic enemas, nasal sprays composed of essential oils. To supplement this, the patient was also given intestinal disinfectants and trace elements and was, of course, prescribed a healthy, natural diet.

This treatment was carried out for six months, until September.

Results as at 20th September 1958:

Weight: gain of 7kg (just over a stone). Tests (full blood count, including estimated sedimentation rate) were normal.

No temperature. Excellent appetite and digestion.

The patient had already resumed his work as a writer two months previously.

In December 1958, nine months after the beginning of the treatment, his general condition was excellent, with a noticeable increase in vitality. he now weighed 88kg (nearly 14 stone) (a gain of 20kg (over 3 stone) in 9 months).

In June 1959, the patient informed me that for the past 3 or 4 months he had been feeling "fit as a fiddle" from the moment he got up every morning.

15 months later, in September 1960, he was in perfect health, was sleeping and eating well and was full of vitality. Weight: 87kg. He still complained of gastric pains, however. X-rays were inconclusive, but suggested the presence of an ulcer.

He was given simple anti-ulcer treatment and drainage of the liver.

In September 1970, 12 years after the start of the treatment, his general condition was excellent.

Apart from aromatic treatments administered on an occasional basis, the patient had been given trace elements, clay, plant extracts to counteract mineral deficiency and packed cell therapy.

Case No 2: Mr P, aged 46 years.

The patient had been suffering from pulmonary tuberculosis since 1941 and had been declared unfit for work in 1943. He had had several stays in sanatoria. Thoracoplasty of 5 ribs performed in 1953.

When examined in 1959, his general condition was poor – weight 62kg ($9\frac{1}{2}$ stone) for a height of 1m 76cm (5 ft 9in).

He was suffering from physical and mental debility, poor appetite and severe hepatism which had, for some years, necessitated a strict diet. He was depressed and anxious and suffered from recurring headaches.

Treatment: Phyto- and aromatherapy, phosphorus, Vitamin D_2, trace elements.

17th April 1959 (one month later): the patient had gained 5kg (11lbs) in weight. He was feeling much stronger and had been free of headaches since the first day of the treatment. He had tried a relatively rich meal containing butter, chocolate and alcohol and had suffered no ill effects whatsoever.

In June 1959, results of blood tests were normal.

In September 1959, his general condition was perfect. The patient was suffering no discomfort at all and his psychological state was excellent once more. He was no longer following a diet and weighed 68kg 500g (11 stone) – a gain of 6kg (a stone) in six months.

The treatment was continued as described above.

In July 1960, this treatment was still producing satisfactory results. In fact, such was the improvement in Mr P's condition that, when jeered at one day by an abattoir worker, he attacked the man, cutting his eyes and upper lip and knocking him out, so that he had to be taken to hospital.

Supplementary point: Mr P, who had a 23-year-old daughter, told us that his wife had become pregnant.

In May 1965, six years after the start of his treatment, he was still in good health and was the father of a fine baby girl.

Senescence
Case No 1: Mr L, aged 68 years.
The patient was suffering from obese senescence and weighed 85kg (13 stone) for a height of 1m 67cm (5ft 6in). For 5 years he had been suffering from physical and mental debility. He was incapable of any activity and spent his days in an armchair, weeping. He also suffered from severe arthrosis and an enlarged prostate. He had an excess of glucose in the blood (1.50g) and his blood pressure was 16/7.

In January 1960 he was treated by phytotherapy and aromatherapy in order to eliminate toxins from the body and to regulate his blood pressure and glucose level. Supplementary treatment: sea-water, phosphorus, magnesium, healthy diet.

Two months later, the patient had undergone a complete transformation, he could walk 3 miles without feeling tired, carry heavy loads and help his wife in the running of her shop. His prostatism was responding to treatment (he no longer suffered from incontinence). He had recovered his spirits and had lost 5kg (11 lbs) in weight.

The results of tests carried out in May 1960, 4 months after the beginning of the treatment, were as follows:
- glucose: 1.20g, instead of 1.50 as in February;
- cholesterol: 2.02g, instead of 2.30g;
- calcium: 91mg, instead of 66mg;
- phosphorus: 44mg as before (normal);
- blood pressure: 14/9 instead of 16/7.

This treatment was continued for 8 months. In February 1962: general condition excellent.

The patient was seen every 3 months and in February 1963 the results of his treatment were still very satisfactory.

Case No 2: Mr S, 65 years of age.
Plethoric senescent: height 1m 72cm (5ft 8in); weight 95kg (about 15 stone). Marked physical and mental debility which had begun a year previously after a violent emotional shock. Neurasthenia, anxiety, insomnia, loss of memory, irritability. An industrialist, this man had reached the stage where he was finding it impossible to continue to run

his large London-based company, and so was seriously considering giving up.

Further symptoms: fortnightly attacks of gout which had occurred for the preceding ten years. Considerable arthrosis. Cramps in upper and lower limbs.

Examination showed hyperglobulinaemia, a cholesterol level of 2.70g, increase in the blood's viscosity with lowering of blood pressure to 13/10 and a rise in the level of alpha 2 globulin (haemogliasis).[4]

Finally, tests revealed hepatic insufficiency. The electrocardiogram tracing was normal.

The patient was given detoxifying phytotherapy and aromatherapy treatment in February 1951. The aim was to improve circulation, combat gout and generally normalise. The following were added: phosphorus and trace elements.

In April 1959 there was marked improvement in the general condition.

It was decided to give *packed cell treatment*. In an organism already at this stage of transformation, such treatment has every chance of producing a thoroughly satisfactory result: placenta, liver, spleen, heart, hypothalamus, testis (14th April 1959).

After a strong reaction of gout in both knees – previously treated by phytotherapy and clay plasters – the results were normal.

In June 1959 his general state of health was excellent. The patient had resumed all his previous activities and had regained the exceptional form which had always been characteristic of him.

April 1961: phyto- and aromatherapy had been continued intermittently since June 1959. The satisfactory results had been maintained. It should be noted that the patient had only three minor crises of gout (in the big toe) in two years, compared to the fortnightly attacks which he had experienced in the preceeding ten.

June 1962: the excellent results were maintained.

June 1963: condition still excellent.

The patient died as the result of an accident in 1965.

Other cases
Case No 1: **Atherosclerosis, haemogliasis.**
This case concerns a man of 64 who in April 1962 showed a disturbing difficulty in reading and speech, together with severe loss of memory.

---

4   Word coined by Dr de Larebeyrette to denote the syndrome which he discovered and has described. This syndrome approximates to the ancient notion of "thick blood". Haemogliasis consists of characteristic disturbance of the blood, together with a greater or lesser degree of debility and disorders of ideation and memory. Blood pressure is normally low.

The patient was overweight – 80kg (12½ stone) for a height of 1m 70cm (5ft 7in) – and for several months previously had complained of persistent fatigue.

Analysis showed an augmented blood viscosity, and a negative cholesterolytic power[5] and a marked rise in alpha 2 globulins – all symptoms of haemogliasis

The patient was treated by phyto- and aromatherapy, sea-water, liver extracts, thyroid trace hormones and iodine.

After 5 months the total cholesterol level had dropped from 2.30g to 2.20g. More importantly, the cholesterolytic power, which had been –13%, was now + 17%. Alpha 2 globulins had fallen from 20% to 13%. The patient had made a perfect physical and mental recovery.

His state of health in November 1965 continued to be excellent.

Case No 2: The after-effects of hemiplegia.

Mrs B, aged 68, suffered hemiplegia (paralysis) of the left side in June 1959. She came to us in September 1960, still exhibiting slight paralysis of the upper left limb and severely lowered mental ability – it was impossible for her to find her words and she suffered from total loss of memory, which prevented her from engaging in any sort of cerebral activity. A recent electroencephalogram showed a "graph of generalised cerebro-vascular damage of arteriosclerotic type".

Ophthalmological examination (Dr D): sclerosis of arteriole type.

The patient was treated by phyto- and aromatherapy, phosphoric acid magnesium, trace elements, Quinton's plasma, fresh cells.

Four months later the paralysis of the upper left limb had disappeared, the patient had begun to read again and her general condition showed continuing, regular improvement.

Up until October 1963, she was seen once every month or every two months, and given the same treatments.

By May 1963 the patient, who had for some time recovered the greater part of her physical and mental powers, was a source of astonishment to her acquaintances. She was able to make long train journeys by herself to attend to her interests in Alsace.

A control electroencephalogram was carried out on 9th April 1963. Taking account of the patient's age, the whole spectrum of cerebral activity appeared spontaneous and normal. There was no durable hemis-

---

5 The cholesterolytic *power* of serum appears to be extremely significant, more so even than the total level of cholesterol in the blood. This power registers the ability of serum, at 37°, to *dissolve* within 36 or 48 hours a certain quantity of crystallised cholesterol added to the serum or to allow it to precipitate either wholly or in part (Loeper and Lemaire).

For the same level of blood cholesterol some patients will produce tissue precipitation, others not.

At the age of 60, 80% of serums are precipitant. This means that (other factors being equal) there is a marked tendency to precipitant conditions: atheroma, coronaritis, lithiasis.

pheric asymmetry and no transitory paroxysmal manifestation. A complete all-round improvement had taken place.

These results were confirmed in July 1965.

Case No. 3: Obesity in an adolescent.

B, a youth aged 16, weighed 85kg (about 13½ stone) for a height of 1m 62 (5ft 4in). The basal metabolic rate had fallen to –6%. Various treatments had been tried without effect, and the boy, like his family, was desperate.

In July 1961 he was treated with phyto- and aromatherapy, thyroid treatment and sea-water. Naturally, bread, cakes, pastries and delicatessen foods were forbidden.

In September 1961 he was given packed cell therapy. Three months later, young B had lost 17kg (more than 2½ stone) in weight.

These results were confirmed in September 1970, no further treatment having been necessary – indeed, the diet had long since been abandoned. At the age of 25 the patient was in perfect health and possessed of Herculean strength. his height was 1m 73cm (5ft 8in) and his weight 74kg (roughly 11½ stone).

Case No. 4: Osteitis.

In 1956 48-year-old Mr B was troubled by a small sore at the tip of his big toe; this led to the removal of an ingrowing toenail. The wound was discharging through a fistula.

Curettage of the consecutive osteitis led to a second fistula.

The first phalange of the toe was amputated in May 1958. A fistula persisted.

The second phalange was amputated in February 1959 (by Professor P). Stubborn suppuration ensued, hindering the healing process.

Professor P then proposed a lumbar sympathectomy[6].

The patient was seen in September 1959.

Clinical condition: suppurating wound at the stump where the left toe had been amputated. Radiologically there was discrete alteration of the antero-internal edge of the cartilage in the first left metatarsal.

The following were normal: urea, glucose level, cholesterol level, keto- and hydroxysteroids, sedimentation rate, prothrombin time, heparin tolerance level, electrocardiogram.

The protidogram, however, showed a high rate of disturbance.

The following treatment was begun: phyto- and aromatherapy, trace elements, magnesium.

---

6   Resection of a greater or lesser length of sympathetic nerve. In this case it was suggested that the part of the sympathetic chain along and behind the lumbar vertebrae be removed.

Since the sympathetic nerve is vaso-constrictive it was hoped that by excising it the blood vessels affected by it would dilate, thus ensuring improved irrigation of the tissue.

Locally, compresses of pure natural essence of lavender were used.

Five months later, in January 1960, the same treatment having been continued in the intervening period, *the wound had totally healed.* Already for a month the patient had been able to wear shoes and walk like anyone else. He then resumed dancing and ski-ing as well.

May 1961: improvement maintained. No therapy whatsoever had been given for a year.

In November 1965, and again in June 1970, examinations showed that the patient was in perfect health and had no need of further treatment.

Case No. 5: **Diabetes**
This concerns a man of 73 who had previously enjoyed perfect health. Since 1959 his glucose level had been 1.98g.

His blood pressure was 19/12. X-rays revealed severe vertebral arthrosis, with distortion of the vertebrae resulting in pressure on the inter-vertebral discs.

There was physical and sexual debility.

Hereditary antecedents: the patient's father and mother had both died of pulmonary tuberculosis.

He was seen in February 1960.

Treatment: phyto- and aromatherapy, and phosphorus; he was also advised to follow a restricted diet.

Two months later, in April 1960, his glucose level was 1.11g and his blood pressure 15/10.

Treatment was continued. Trace elements "zinc-nickel-cobalt" were added.

The glucose level changed as follows:

June	1.41g
July	1.22g
September	1.30g
November	1.24g
January 1961	1.09g

The patient achieved an astonishing level of vitality. His sexual drive by which he set great store was regained. His blood pressure was 14/9.

June 1963: glucose level 1.12g, condition excellent.

December 1972: at 86, Mr B may be bowed by age, but he still acts as mayor of his village.

Case No. 6:
Mrs P, from the Dordogne, became *depressed* to an alarming degree in March 1958 when her grandson joined the army in Algeria. In the space of a few weeks this vivacious, outgoing woman was no more than a shadow of herself. She no longer remembered anything and shortly thereafter lost her reason. Thinking she was going outdoors she would bury

herself in a cupboard and remain there. After clearing the table she would take the washing-up to the bathroom.

Her son-in-law was anxious to try everything in his power to help, since she had been a good mother-in-law.

I treated her by phyto- and aromatherapy, with phosphorus and trace elements. I brought her to Paris to give her packed cell treatment: liver, spleen, anterior hypothalamus, pituitary gland.

After two months, Mrs P seemed ten years younger. She was in excellent physical and mental health.

This improved state lasted for $2\frac{1}{2}$ years. Then, in December 1960 returning home on foot to her house in Vézac, she took a short cut and fell into a frozen pond. A farmworker heard her cries and dragged her out only just in time, but the physical shock and terrible fear that she was going to drown took their toll.

That very evening the pattern of March 1958 reasserted itself.

I advised that the woman be brought to Paris for further packed cell treatment, This was given on 6th December 1960. The treatment was completed by administering plants and essences.

Six weeks later Mrs P had recovered. In 1970, that is six years later, she was still well at the age of 83. Mrs P takes no medication other than occasional herbal infusions. Some are prescribed, others she makes herself, for she has the countrywoman's knowledge of herbs.

Case No. 7: **Chlorosis**
Chlorosis is a kind of anaemia which only affects young women and for some time past it has been extremely difficult to find a case.

In 1962 I was presented with a genuine case. The patient was a pale, thin, tired girl who had not had a menstrual period for about 6 months. Analysis had produced no real clue except a red blood count of 3,900,000.

She was treated with plants (tinctures and powders), aromatic essences (pine needles, thyme, lavender, geranium, clove, eucalyptus, lemon), phosphoric acid and iodine. I had no worries about her diet since she was in the care of a family who were fully aware of the importance of proper nourishment.

After 4 months the red blood count had increased to 4,760,000. Menstrual function returned after 2 months. In 4 months the patient put on 6kg (over 13lbs) in weight.

In 1970 the patient was not only well but had married. Natural hormones cured the chlorosis. They even enabled the woman to give birth to a fine baby.

Case No. 8: **Complete physiological distress**
Mrs H, aged 50, was a former victim of Ravensbrück concentration camp where she had experienced many forms of maltreatment: experi-

mental injections of unknown substances, beatings . . . the reader may draw up his own list.

When seen in 1960 her health was precarious. She had the appearance of an old woman: her skin was wrinkled, she walked bent up. She weighed 47kg (roughly 7½ stone) for a height of 1m 58 (5ft 3½ in).

The patient complained of an extreme lassitude which she had experienced ever since she had been repatriated in 1944. She suffered from loss of appetite and insomnia.

She experienced generalised vertebral pain. X-rays showed osteoporosis throughout the spine, dorso-lumbar scoliosis and numerous displaced and rotated vertebrae (cervical, dorsal and lumbar).

There was a further, rather curious, symptom: clinical and radiological examination showed a reduction of the lower maxilla, together with contraction of the bones of the foot (her feet had become a whole shoe-size smaller).

Mrs H complained of generalised aches and pains in her bones. She had not been able to wear a pair of shoes for many years.

Finally, she had not had a menstrual period since 1944, when she had been the subject of German medical experiment.

Her psychological state was frightening: she suffered from a deep-rooted instability, anxiety, crises of excitement and of despair. She had totally lost her memory.

She had undergone numerous forms of treatment, with little real success.

Tests indicated severe damage.

This patient was treated with phyto- and aromatherapy, magnesium and fresh cells.

A month after the start of treatment she regained her appetite and ability to sleep. Her skin and features grew visibly younger. The pain in her vertebrae disappeared. Her memory partially returned. For the first time in years she was able to read without glasses. Her psychological state improved vastly: she became calm yet lively, and her nightmares stopped.

Further tests done as a control showed a remarkable transformation, five months after the start of treatment. They showed that she was now, by and large, normal.

She put on 6kg (13¼ lbs) in weight. For the first time in years she found she could wear high-heeled shoes. She was able to drive herself about in her own car.

September 1961 saw her condition consolidated. She had ceased treatment three months earlier.

In December 1974 her condition is excellent – thanks to occasional treatment with herbs and aromatherapy.

Since publication of the first edition of this book in 1964, a number of doctors have been able to observe similar cases of their own, using these methods. One such doctor has undertaken a number of experiments in the realm of *psychiatry*. I have set out some of his observations below. The reader will find yet again the favourable results to which aromatic essences, plants and various forms of biological therapy have made him familiar. But the special interest of these studies lies in the fact that they concern, on the one hand, patients with *chronic mental conditions*, many of whom had been hospitalised for a considerable number of years, and, on the other, patients who had undergone only limited psychiatric treatment but who had been treated with *synthetic drugs*.

In the first category, the severe nature of the mental affliction rules out any *simulation*. In the second, the patients had often been treated by a varying number of doctors of "classical" persuasion and had as a result arrived at a state of permanent *frustration* with current orthodox medicine.

In both cases, reaction to natural therapy was comparable to that of "normal" patients.

Case No. 1:

Mrs B, aged 49, suffered from serious nervous depression. In trying to commit suicide by jumping out of a window she had broken her pelvis, and on another occasion both her wrists.

In October 1969 the patient was confined to bed with the onset of ankylosis, locking of the neck and lack of power in the upper right limb. She had bedsores on the heels and buttocks.

Psychiatric treatment improved her mental state in a few weeks, but had no effect on her inability to function physically.

In January 1970 she was treated to ease the contractures with thrice-weekly sub-cutaneous and intradermal injections of bidistilled water round the blocked joints and in the muscles, and in addition she was massaged with aromatic liniment.

Her neck became unlocked in a matter of days. The patient cried aloud at the miracle; she was able to move almost normally.

The treatment thereafter consisted of drainage and the making good of mineral deficiency using aromatic plants (tinctures, powdered horsetail, mixtures containing the essences of thyme, lavender, sage, juniper, rosemary) and magnesium; to these were added friction rubs with aromatic substances and generalised baths combining seaweed and aromatic essences.

In three months excellent progress was made both physically and psychologically. The surgeon was astonished at this total recovery and the patient was able to return to her former life.

Case No. 2:

Mrs C was 36 years old. She had been confined to hospital for 6 years, suffering from dementia praecox. Violent and dangerous, this patient also had a chronic bronchial infection and, periodically, an infection of the urinary tract as well. There were periods when she became alarm ingly thin, with a high temperature.

She was treated in December 1969 with "copper-gold-silver" and "manganese-copper", as well as aromatherapy and phytotherapy.

Within ten days her temperature was stabilised at 37°C. There was progressive consolidation of her general condition, her weight increased and she became more active. Her psychological condition was favourably altered.

This progress was seen to have been maintained, nine months later, by regular treatment of a similar nature.

Case No. 3:
Mrs F, aged 56, suffered from deep-seated delirious madness. She had been in hospital for many years.

She had previously had tuberculosis and had suffered for three years from a rhino-pharyngeal infection and chronic bronchitis with persistent fever which resisted antibiotic treatment. Her general condition was poor.

In October 1969 she was treated with trace elements and aromatherapy, both internally and by means of suppositories.

Her temperature became normal in 3 weeks. These results were consolidated by 20 days' treatments each month for 6 months.

Case No. 4:
Mrs M suffered from feverish dementia and had been in hospital for 5 years.

She suffered from vaginal haemorrhaging following an operation for the removal of a benign cyst. Her temperature ranged between 35° and 38°C and she was resistant to antibiotics. Otherwise, clinical and laboratory examination revealed no disorder, apart from signs of infection of the blood.

This syndrome of unexplained, fluctuating fever with neither clinical nor biological indication of its origin is frequently found amongst psychiatric patients. The reason is thought to lie in the medicinal poisoning which these chronic patients experience and a concomitant breaking down of the natural defence barriers. In this altered state, the organism is prey to a multiplicity of minor infections (broncho-pulmonary, genitourinary or intestinal), or infections which it is hard to localise.

Anti-infection treatment by aromatherapy in this case normalised the temperature in 15 days (December 1968).

Three months later there was an attack of fever caused by chronic bronchitis.

The following aromatic treatment was given intra-muscularly and orally: thyme, rosemary, sage, cinnamon, eucalyptus and camomile, backed up by trace elements. The patient was cured within a week.

Fourteen months later, these results were found to have been maintained with simple, analogous back-up treatment from time to time.

Case No. 5:
Miss H, aged 55, was debilitised.

She had had a chronic infection of the urinary tract for a number of years: colibacillosis, bloody urine, highly painful cystitis.

In March 1970 there was a sudden intensifying of the condition, fever, and a general state of prostration.

Treatment by phyto- and aromatherapy and phosphoric acid (as acidifier) sedated the symptoms within a fortnight. The patient was able to get up again.

The results were confirmed after a further 4 months of continuing treatment.

Case No. 6:
Mrs P, aged 66, suffered from hallucinatory psychosis.

In January 1970 she had influenza with a temperature of 38–39°C and abundant expectoration. Blood tests showed considerable disorder.

She was treated with antibiotics for 3 days and then aromatherapy (essential oils of thyme, pine, juniper, rosemary and eucalyptus), "copper-gold-silver", magnesium and powdered horsetail.

General recovery and renewal of activity in two weeks.

Case No. 7:
Mrs R, aged 36, suffered from nervous depression. She had already experienced a number of physiological misfortunes (e.g. cranial traumatism, removal of the uterus).

Confined to her bed, the patient complained of vertebral pain especially in the lumbar region and the right shoulder. She also suffered from persistent cystitis.

In November 1969 she was treated with a special phytotherapeutic preparation and by aromatherapy: also with injectable extracts of freeze-dried kidney and oral vaccine.

Externally, she was given massage using aromatic liniment; also baths combining seaweed and aromatic essences.

There was considerable improvement after 6 days and the patient was able to get up for the first time.

After two months the patient was able to leave the hospital. She continued to follow a course of treatment, both internal and external, by aromatherapy, drainage using plants (artichoke, ash leaves, blackcurrant leaves and horsetail) and sulphur.

Her urine was normal.

With patients who have experienced *profound alteration of the psyche*, there can be no fear of simulation. These people have been helped or cured without knowing the why or the wherefore. But those who are in daily contact with them and care for them have indeed been astonished at the changes.

There was no real need for these additional examples in order to be convinced of the positive effects of therapy using natural extracts.

What is important to remember here is that the cases concern organisms which have been poisoned by long-term, high-dose chemotherapy – which, it should be said, is sometimes unavoidable given the complexity of the psychological condition.

Aromatherapy and plant and biological therapies have confirmed beyond doubt the effects, sometimes unsurpassed, of which they are capable.

As regards the type of patient who (and this is a category which is growing all the time), while being "abnormal", is not *totally* "closed" and unreceptive, one should perhaps consider the therapeutic link established between the patient and physician by this sort of treatment. The result of explaining to a patient the effect which natural treatments can have is to awaken in him some sort of interest – of the kind accorded a "new" medicine in any case, but perhaps with a bonus because it involves a "human" approach. This has the advantage of being, in Dr Henri Ey's phrase, "a beneficial encounter, an awakening of consciousness and the *beginning of a return to vitality*".

A great many chapters could be filled with many more case histories: I have for my part published significant numbers of cases in my various works, most of which have been selected from those where chemotherapy has failed. The results which have been achieved prove that doctors would often do better to administer natural medications initially, and be prepared to add this or that synthetic medicine where necessity demanded. For if chemotherapy sometimes produces results which phyto-aromatherapy would be unable to achieve, the opposite is also and much more often true, as the facts abundantly demonstrate.

6. Some Formulae for Medicinal Wines and Vinegars, Elixirs and Compound Preparations

By way of illustration, I thought it would be interesting to pick out a few of the many hundreds of formulae. It is not question of drawing up a complete list but only of showing the kind of weapons our predecessors used in their war against illness.

Some Medicinal Wines

Cinnamon wine or cordial:

cinnamon	30g
Malaga wine	500g

Leave to macerate for 6 days, then filter.

What our ancestors called "Hippocras" (Vinum hippocraticum) was wine aromatised with cinnamon.

Prepare cascarilla, juniper and ginger wines in the same way.

Bitter diuretic wine (Corvisart):

powdered cinchona bark	
pleurisy root	30g of each
angelica	
squill	
juniper	10g of each
mace	
wormwood	
melissa (balm)	2g of each
lemon rind	
winter's bark	60g of each
alcohol at 34°	
white wine	4 litres

Steep the crushed plants for 24 hours. Force through a sieve, then filter through paper.

Begin with 4 tablespoonfuls a day, increasing the dose gradually. To treat debility of the digestive organs.

A wine to combat leucorrhoea:

cinchona bark	180g
calamus	45g
quassia	24g
cinnamon	24g
elder	24g
alcohol	1,500g
pure water	9 litres

After macerating sufficiently, sieve, then add:

tincture of mars	375g
orange-blossom water	750g
sugar syrup	180g

60g first thing in the morning, in cases of *leucorrhoea*.

Aromatic wine:

vulnerary spirit	125g
red wine	875g

Mix. Filter after 2 days.

aromatic plants (compounds)	100g
vulnerary tincture	100g
red wine	875g

Allow the aromatic compounds to steep for 10 days in the wine. Force through a sieve, add the spirit and filter.

This was widely used in the past in fermentations or *vaginal douches*.

Bitter aromatic wine (compound vermouth, tonic wine):

1 –	gentian	85g
	centaury	56g
	orange peel	42g
	wormwood	56g

2 –	calamus	85g
	elecampane	85g
	galangal	42g
	lesser wormwood	28g
	clary sage	28g
	iris	28g

3 –	yellow cinchona	28g

4 –	coriander	85g
	cinnamon	14g
	clove	7g
	nutmegs	3

Make 4 separate sachets, put them at the bottom of a 50-litre barrel and fill the barrel with unfermented wine. When fermentation is finished, decant.

Formerly used as a stomachic to counteract sluggish and painful digestion *in those of weak health.*

Compound cinnamon wine (Hippocras, hippocratic wine, cordial wine):

sweet almonds	125g
cinnamon	45g
sugar	900g
brandy	360g
Madeira wine	720g

Steep for a few days. To the strained liquid add:

musk	} 0.09g of each
ambergis	

Another formula:.

cinnamon	7.50g
ginger	1.00g
nutmeg	0.50g
clove	0.50g
lesser cardamine	0.25g
zest of bitter oranges	25g
alcohol	25.00g
simple syrup	150.00g
a generous red wine	1 litre

Compound senna wine:

senna	120g
coriander (seeds)	8g
fennel (seeds)	8g
sherry	1 litre

Macerate the crushed plants for 3 days. Filter. Add 90g of raisins, macerate for 24 hours. Filter again.

From 60 to 100g to be taken in the morning on an empty stomach as a laxitive and carminative, in cases of *flatulent dyspepsia.*

Purgative tonic wine:

senna pods	30g
crushed rhubarb	24g
cloves	4g
saffron	4g
sherry	1 litre

Macerate for 6 days, stirring frequently, and filter. Two or three spoonfuls of this wine act as a *tonic* and five or six spoonfuls produce a *laxative* effect.

Some Medicinal Vinegars

Antiseptic vinegar or "Vinegar of the Four Thieves" (Marseilles vinegar):

greater wormwood	40g
lesser wormwood	40g
rosemary	40g
sage	40g
mint	40g
rue	40g
lavender	40g
calamus	5g
cinnamon	5g
clove	5g
nutmeg	5g
garlic	5g
camphor	10g
crystallised acetic acid	40g
white vinegar	2,500g

Steep the plants in the vinegar for 10 days. Force through a sieve. Add the camphor dissolved in the acetic acid, then filter.

This vinegar finds its use in the prevention of *contagious diseases*. Rub it on face and hands and burn it in the room. It can also be kept in small bottles for the vapours to be sniffed in cases of fainting.

The story goes that this formula was revealed in the 17th century by four corpse-robbers caught red-handed during the time of the great plagues of Toulouse (1628–1631). Their disregard for the contagion thoroughly astonished the judges ... The archives of the Parliament of Toulouse record that: "During the great plague, four robbers were convicted of going to the houses of plague-victims, strangling them in their beds and then looting their dwellings: for this they were condemned to be burned at the stake, and in order to have the sentence mitigated they revealed their secret preservative; after which they were hanged."

The original recipe in fact was as follows:
- 3 pints of strong white wine vinegar
- a handful each of wormwood, meadowsweet, juniper berries, wild marjoram and sage
- 50 cloves
- 2 ounces of elecampane root
- 2 ounces of angelica
- 2 ounces of rosemary
- 2 ounces of horehound
- 3g camphor

244

Aromatic and antiseptic vinegar:

spirit of melissa (balm)	15g
essence of clove	4g
lemon essence	10g
lavender essence	10g
white vinegar	60g

Mix and filter. Diluted with water, it is used in lotions for the *pruritis* (itching) which accompanies certain skin diseases.

Vinegar mouth-wash or dentifrice:.

pyrethrum root	60g
fine cinnamon	8g
clove	8g
scurvy-grass spirit	60g
red vulnerary water	125g
gum guaiacum	8g
white vinegar	2 litres

Crush the solid ingredients and steep in the vinegar. Meanwhile, dissolve the gum guaiacum in the vulnerary water and scurvy-grass spirit. Add this tincture to the filtered vinegar (the mixture will become cloudy, but will clear in a few days).

Vinegar skin lotion:

alcohol	⎫
strong vinegar	⎬ in equal parts
benzoin	⎭

Leave to macerate. Filter. A few drops added to water will make it milky, at the same time giving it a pleasant perfume and *tonic* properties for the *skin.*

Aromatic English vinegar (smelling salts):

solid acetic acid	250g
camphor	60g
essential oil of lavender	0.50g
essential oil of clove	2g
essential oil of cinnamon	1g

Table vinegar (Maille):

elder flowers	250g
tarragon	375g
water mint	125g
basil	100g
marguerite	100g
savory	100g
thyme	1 pinch

```
bay (leaves) ..................................... 4 or 5
shallot.......................................... 125g
garlic........................................... 31g
cloves .......................................... 40g
cinnamon........................................ 40g
ripe pimento .................................... 6g
chervil ......................................... 180g
ground pepper................................... 60g
salt, spring onions............................. to taste
the strongest Orleans vinegar ................... 3 litres
```

Put ingredients into an earthenware jar sealed with parchment and leave for six weeks exposed to sunlight. Filter and put into sealed bottles.

Some Elixirs

Anti-gout elixir:
```
grey cinchona ................................... 125g
red poppy....................................... 60g
sassafras ....................................... 30g
rum............................................. 5 litres
```
Steep for two weeks, then strain and add:
```
guaiacum root................................... 60g
```
Steep for a further two weeks, then add a syrup made from:
```
sarsaparilla .................................... 125g
sugar........................................... 1,250g
```
1 or 2 tablespoonfuls 2 or 3 times a day.

Chaussier's antiseptic elixir:
```
cinchona ........................................ 64g
cascarilla ....................................... 16g
saffron ......................................... 2g
Spanish wine.................................... 500g
cinnamon........................................ 12g
brandy ......................................... 500g
```
Steep for several days, strain and add:
```
sugar........................................... 150g
sulphuric ether ................................. 6g
```
This elixir was used in the typhus outbreak of 1814–1815.

Elixir for venereal disease:
```
gum guaiacum................................... 220g
sassafras ....................................... 155g
balsam of Peru ................................. 15g
alcohol ......................................... 1,250g
```
One teaspoonful in a glass of sugared water (gout, *syphilis*).

Elixir mouthwash or dentifrice:

essence of Ceylon cinnamon	1g
essence of Chinese aniseed	2g
essence of cloves	2g
essence of peppermint	8g
tincture of benzoin	8g
tincture of cochineal	20g
tincture of guaiacum	8g
tincture of pyrethrum	8g
alcohol at 80°	1,000g

Mix. Filter after 24 hours.

Half a teaspoonful in a glass of warm water.

Another elixir mouthwash:

guaiacum spirits	187g
camphorated spirits	4g
essence of peppermint	6 drops
essence of scurvy-grass	6 drops
essence of rosemary	6 drops

Odontalgic elixir:

guaiacum	15g
pyrethrum	4g
nutmeg	4g
clove	2g
essence of rosemary	10 drops
essence of bergamot	4 drops
alcohol at 70°	100g

Leave to steep for 8 days. Filter. One teaspoonful in a glass of water, in mouthwashes (toothache).

Grande-Chartreuse elixir:

fresh melissa (balm)	640g
fresh hyssop	640g
fresh angelica	320g
cinnamon	160g
saffron	40g
mace	10g

After macerating for 8 days in 10 litres of alcohol, express and distil on to a quantity of fresh plants: melissa, hyssop. After some time add 1,250g of sugar and filter.

Another formula:

essence of lemon balm	2g
essence of hyssop	2g

247

```
essence of angelica .............................. 10g
essence of peppermint ........................... 20g
essence of nutmeg................................. 2g
essence of cloves ................................ 2g
alcohol at 80°............................... 2 litres
sugar....................................... to taste
```

May be coloured yelllow with a few drops of tincture of saffron, and green with a few drops of indigo in solution or alcoholic tincture of elder leaves.

Some Compound Preparations

The term "compounds" is applied to mixtures of a number of plants, or parts of plants which have been chopped or crushed. Compounds are used in making infusions, macerations and decoctions for internal or external use.

Antispasmodic compounds:
```
valerian ...................................... 90g
orange leaves ................................. 60g
yarrow ........................................ 30g
```

Another formula:
```
lavender....................................... 50g
melissa (balm)................................ 100g
basil ........................................ 100g
catmint....................................... 100g
```
As an infusion for *convulsive "whooping" coughs.*

Aromatic compounds:
```
sage leaves ...............................  ⎫
thyme leaves ..............................  ⎪
wild thyme leaves..........................  ⎪
rosemary leaves............................  ⎬  in equal parts
hyssop leaves..............................  ⎪
origanum leaves ...........................  ⎪
wormwood leaves............................  ⎪
mint leaves................................  ⎭
```
In baths or lotions. Infuse in the proportion of 50g to 1 litre of water.

Carminative compounds or seeds (the four "hot" seeds):
```
aniseed....................................  ⎫
fennel ....................................  ⎬  equal  quantities
coriander .................................  ⎪
caraway ...................................  ⎭
```
For flatulence.

Diuretic compounds:

dried fennel roots	
dried roots of butcher's-broom	
dried roots of wild celery	equal quantities
dried parsley roots	
dried asparagus roots	

As an infusion: 20g to a litre of water.
(This forms the basis of the "syrup of the 5 roots": 3 to 5 tablespoonfuls a day.)

Compounds for smoking (Trousseau):

stramonium	30g
sage	15g

Divide into 20 cigarettes or smoke in a pipe: for *asthma.*

Vermifuge compounds for enemas:

wormwood	30g
valerian	30g
tansy seeds	15g
orange peel	15g

Two tablespoonfuls to $\frac{1}{2}$ litre of boiling water. Leave to infuse for 10 minutes. Strain. This quantity is sufficient for two enemas, to each of which should be added a spoonful of oil (threadworm and whip-worm).

SOME ADDITIONAL USEFUL FORMULAE

***"Climarome"** (proprietary medicament):
a mixture of the essences of lavender, niaouli, pine, mint and thyme.

Introduced recently, this product is not a medicine in the proper meaning of the term; but the essences of which it is composed combine their *antiseptic* and *aromatic* virtues to *protect* the respiratory passages in the same way as do pine forests and fields of lavender and thyme.[1].

20 drops on a handkerchief, to be inhaled several times a day.

***"Tégarome"** (proprietary medicament):
a mixture based on the essences of lavender, thyme, sage, eucalyptus, rosemary and cypress.[1]

For the treatment of: sunstroke, first and second degree burns (not extensive), insect bites and stings (wasps, spiders, mosquitos, etc), cuts, spots and pimples of certain kinds, bruises; also for oral hygiene.

According to the type of case it should be applied either neat, or diluted in warm water in compresses (50 drops to a glass) or mouthwashes and gargles (20 drops to a glass).

Experience has also shown that this product may be used, neat or in compresses, in local applications for shingles. We have not yet recorded

1   Phyto-East, 6 rue des Cigognes, 67000 Strasbourg.

a single failure in 25 years among countless cases treated within the first 15–20 days in this way. As an added safeguard, the treatment includes magnesium administered orally. The cure is effected within 5 and 8 days.

There is no doubt that the beneficial effect of **Tégarome** is such cases is due to the antiviral and cicatrising properties of some of the essences included in its formula.

*Aromatic tincture of arnica:

                arnica flowers 50g
                clove.................................... 10g
                cinnamon................................ 10g
                ginger 10g
                aniseed................................. 100g
                alcohol .... 1 litre

Macerate for 8 days. Strain.

1 spoonful in half a glass of honey water, repeated 2 or 3 times a day, in the case of a *fall* or *bruising*. Good for *toothache*.

*Miracle water:

                angelica 30g
                rosemary 30g
                marjoram................................ 30g
                costmary 30g
                hyssop 30g
                wormwood................................ 30g
                mint 30g
                thyme................................... 30g
                sage.................................... 45g
                brandy .... 2½ litres

Put into a bottle and leave exposed to sunlight for 15 days. Filter. Decant into bottles and cork.

To treat: indigestion, constipation, intestinal infections, debility, vertigo. 1 teaspoon each morning.

As a dressing for wounds, sores and abscesses, use in compresses (changed 2 or 3 times a day).

Opodeldoch balsam:

Melt in a glass vessel in a bain-marie:

                grated animal-fat soap .... 30g, with
                alcohol at 90°.......................... 250g

Add:

                powdered camphor 24g
                essential oil of thyme 2g
                essential oil of rosemary 6g

Pour into jars while still hot; the mixture congeals on cooling.

(As a friction rub for rheumatic pains).

And for sexual deficiencies, it is always worth trying:
Italian essence:

cinnamon	90g
greater cardamom	60g
galangal	60g
clove	15g
long pepper	12g
nutmeg	8g
ambergris	0.2g
musk	0.2g
alcohol at 90°	1 litre

Leave to macerate for a month, then filter.
(*Aphrodisiac:* 20 to 30 drops on a sugar-lump . . . I guarantee results.)

7.   How to Gather and Preserve Aromatic Plants

Aromatic essences in therapeutic use are generally given in the form of drops or pills. But we treat ourselves no less every day by using aromatics in cooking; or we may equally well look after our health by taking infusions of aromatic plants.

For this reason I thought it helpful to give some information on the gathering and preserving of plants, together with dosages for infusions and decoctions.

The therapeutic effectiveness of the plants depends very much on the way they are gathered and dried, for it is vital that they conserve their active constituents to the fullest extent.

To make sure of this, they should be dried in the sun, in a loft, in the oven or in a drying cupboard.

The flowers should be protected from light, heat and damp. Plants are best preserved on racks or suspended in small packets. All foreign matter, and dead or damaged parts, should be removed beforehand.

As a general rule, roots should be dried in a dry atmosphere and stored away from the damp. Mucilaginous roots should be dried in the oven. Bark and wood are best dried in the sun or in a drying cupboard, and should also be kept in a dry place.

Flowers, leaves and seeds must be dried in the shade, in a barn or room with a dry atmosphere. They should be stored in boxes and in a dry place.

Plants should be gathered in dry weather once the sun has risen and the dew cleared.

Flowers should be picked before they have fully bloomed. Roses and pinks should be picked as buds.

The leaves too are gathered before they are fully developed, certainly no later than the moment the flower buds begin forming (apart from those plants whose leaves or flowering tops are used on their own, e.g. the Labiatae).

Buds should be gathered in the spring, fruit in the autumn, roots in spring and autumn, tree-bark in winter, the bark of shrubs in autumn and the bark of resin-bearing trees in the spring.

If plant therapy has fallen into disrepute, then neglect of these rules has been a major cause.

Using Plants in Infusions or Decoctions

Plants are given in the same dose whether fresh or dried; fresh plants are heavier and their principles more active.
- one pinch correspondes to 2 to 3g,
- one dessertspoonful to 5g,
- one tablespoon equals 10g,
- one handful about 30 or 40g.

Unless otherwise stated, the quantities are for adults. For children, prepare in the same way and then dilute as follows:
- at 1 year old: 1 part infusion to 4 of water.
- 1–3 years: 2 parts infusion to 3 of water.
- 3–5 years: 3 parts infusion to 2 of water.
- 5–10 years: 4 parts infusion to 1 of water.

When treating adults – and of course, more especially, children – individual susceptibilities sometimes have to be taken into account.

When boiling is required, the plants should be placed in cold water and then brought to the boil.

It is best to drink the infusions unsweetened; or if sweetened, then with honey rather than sugar.

If no specific time is given, the expression "give one boil" signifies boiling for a few seconds, then removing from the heat and leaving to infuse as directed.

As a general rule, roots, stalks and bark should be boiled for from 5 to 10 minutes.

"One boil" is the correct method for whole plants, leaves, seeds and flowering tops.

Flowers are infused (i.e. boiling water is poured on them).

You are advised to use enamel pans rather than receptacles of bare metal.

All other utensils used should be either made of glass or wood.

Definitions of the Various Methods of Preparing Plants, and their Uses

In this section you will find references to substances whose nature differs from that of the essences. This is because it seemed to me, on balance, to make up a useful collection of information which it would be inappropriate to cut.

Alcoholic tincture: liquid obtained when a fresh plant is kept in alcohol for some considerable time; more specifically, in a quantity of alcohol 5 times the weight of the plant(s).

Aromatic baths: Put 500g aromatic compounds (q.v.) into a sachet (250g for children). Pour on 3 or 4 litres of boiling water and leave to infuse for 10–15 minutes in a covered vessel. Then add to the bath. Here is a guide to the indications of the different herbs, etc:

1 – *juniper:* recommended for arthritis and rheumatism.
2 – *lavender:* sedative (for nervous complaints and insomnia). Indicated also for delicate or run-down children. Alternate with baths of pine, rosemary and seaweed.
3 – *marjoram:* tonic (similar to baths of thyme).
4 – *pine:* also fortifying. Recommended too for rheumatism and gout (local baths may be used to treat excessive sweating of the feet).
5 – *rosemary:* fortifying, especially for children. Also beneficial in cases of rheumatism and weak eyesight.
6 – *sage:* fortifying, for children affected by debility, rickets or scrofula. Beneficial in cases of rheumatism.
7 – *thyme:* again fortifying and, in addition, indicated in cases of arthritis, rheumatism, gout and chronic pulmonary conditions.
8 – *turpentine:* antirheumatic.

Aromatised water: aromatised distilled water (e.g. aromatised or distilled orange-flower water).

Baths of combined essences and seaweed: the recent idea of combining in the same bath both seaweeds of certain types and selected aromatic compounds has, by giving the body the benefit of their different properties, extended the range of indications considerably. We may include here obesity, cellulitis, lymphatism, prolonged convalescence, anaemia, chronic rheumatism, poor circulation, states of demineralisation, premature ageing, menopausal problems, problems of normal ageing and certain skin conditions.

Compounds: the terms given to essences or plants sharing the same properties (e.g. diuretic compounds, sudorific compounds, etc).

Decoction: solution obtained by prolonged boiling of a plant (in a covered vessel). The plant is put in cold water, brought to the boil and boiled for from 10 to 20 minutes. Bark and roots require longer boiling than stems and leaves.

Embrocation: sprinkling a part of the body with an appropriate liquid which is then rubbed into the skin.

Enema (soothing) for diarrhoea, rectitis, piles:

        linseed 15g
        leaves of great mullein 150g
        boiling water 500g

255

Leave to infuse until the water is lukewarm. Forced through a sieve and add the yolk of one egg. Administer half at a time.

Alternatively:
>   poppy heads without seeds 20g
>   boiling water 500g

Leave to infuse for 2 hours, then add 10g of powdered starch.

Alternatively:
>   5 spoonfuls of vinegar
>   400g of warm water

Extract: substance obtained by partial evaporation of an aqueous, alcoholic or ethereal solution of a plant.

Fluid extract: liquid obtained by treating a drug with several times its own weight of water or alcohol and evaporating the result until its weight equals that of the drug used.

Fomentation: application of a heated liquid, either by hand or with the aid of a sponge, brush or flannel.

Friction rub: embrocation.

Fumigation, Dry: burn one or more plants over glowing embers.

Fumigation, Moist: the aromatic vapour obtained by boiling one or more plants in water.

Infusion: the solution obtained by subjecting a plant to the action of boiling water for a few minutes (from 5 to 15 minutes, depending on the plant).

Intract: special extract only obtainable from a plant which has preserved its original composition.

Juices, see Plant Juices.

Laudanum: alcoholic tincture of opium and saffron. Sydenham's laudanum has strength of 10% that of opium and 1% that of morphine (20 drops = 5cg opium. One poppy-head contains 5–6g opium).

Liquid extract, see Fluid extract.

Lotion: boil one or more plants in water and pass through fine muslin; used in washes.

Maceration: solution obtained by steeping a plant in cold water, wine, alcohol or oil to extract its soluble principles. This may take a few hours or several days, sometimes several weeks, depending on the case.

Mustard compress: dip a piece of gauze in warm water, squeeze it out and spread on a flat surface. Sprinkle over it a layer of mustard powder. Apply to the affected part and leave in a place for about ten minutes from the moment the patient begins to feel it smarting.

Mustard plaster, see Sinapism.

Oils: half fill a wide-mouthed jar with dried plants or crushed roots and top up with oil. Allow to macerate for 3 weeks at a mild temperature, stirring from time to time. Decant into a flask. Obtained in this manner are the following medicinal or culinary oils:

>   Camomile oil: used in friction rubs for aches and pains.
>   Oil of St John's wort: for pains and burns.
>   Oil of thyme, bay and rosemary: for grilling meat.

Ointment: preparation for external use, generally consisting of a greasy base (oil, fat) with or without active principles.

Oleo-saccharum: a mixture of essential oils and sugar, used to aromatise drinks.

Plant Juices:

Juice of bitter and aperitive plants (biliary complaints):

>   angelica (green stems) .... 1 small handful
>   fumitory.............................. 2 large handsful
>   wild pansy .... 2 large handsful
>   chicory............................... 2 large handsful
>   dandelion............................. 2 large handsful

Juice of bitter and tonic plants (debility):

>   peppermint .... 1 small handful
>   speedwell............................. 2 large handsful
>   lesser centaury........................ 2 large handsful
>   marsh trefoil .... 2 large handsful
>   hops (green stems) .... 2 large handsful

Juice of antiscorbutic plants (scurvy – mouth ulcers):

>   scurvy-grass.......................... 3 handsful
>   shepherd's-purse....................... 2 handsful
>   watercress .... 3 handsful

Juice of refreshing plants (diuretic):

purslane	1 handful
sorrel	1 handful
lettuce	1 handful
white beet	1 handful
viper's grass (black salsify)	1 handful
dandelion	1 handful

Plaster: adhesive preparation for external use. There are various kinds, distinguished according to their method of manufacture and the material used, e.g. lard, wax, oil, resin.

Rob: a sudorific and depurative syrup.

Sinapism (Mustard plaster): a mixture of mustard powder and water which is applied to the skin as a poultice to provoke a counter-irritation.

Simple syrup: a compound obtained by dissolving 180g sugar in 100g hot or cold water. Therapeutic ingredients are incorporated as required.

Soft extract: see Fluid extract. Evaporation is stopped at the point when the product has the consistency of honey.

Spirit (of aromatic plants): liquid obtained by distilling alcohol on a plant.

Tincture: liquid obtained by dissolving the active constituents of medicinal substances in a suitable liquid (e.g. water, alcohol, ether).

8. Conclusions

> "The sole and constant aim of scientific research should be the understanding of phenomena. The researcher should not have to ask himself if any practical conclusions may be deduced from his observations."
> (Charles Richet).

There always comes a moment when, however disjointed it may have seemed, scientific research lets us perceive the links which will harness it to practical and beneficial ends.

The empirical belief in the therapeutic value of essences seems to us – in the light of the great variety of present-day research – to have been given undeniable substance and astonishing objective proof.

According to F. Decaux,[1] present studies are sufficient to prove that "to the authenticity of its traditional reputation phytotherapy has added more practical claims to be considered a method of therapy relevant today, as much by reason of the discovery and use of a number of new drugs of plant origin as in the extent and variety of their application in pathology".

From the point of view of antisepsis, to take one example, it is surprising to note the disfavour which has dogged aromatherapy through the decades which separate us from the initial work of Chamberland in 1887. Doubtless the competition provided by the concurrent development of chemical antiseptics, such as the hypochlorites and peroxide of hydrogen, can explain the paradox.

As Henri Poincaré said, to doubt everything and to believe everything are two equally comfortable solutions which relieve us of the need to think.

Generally speaking, men are content to scorn what they cannot understand. Well, "it is a wise philosophy not to deny facts simply because they are opposed to our ideas or theories, but rather to seek to verify them".[2]

1   F. Decaux: *Pérennité de la Phytothérapie* – Gazette Médicale (1963).
2   Gazette Médicale (1833).

Which is exactly what has happened in the field of plant essences – which provide the doctor with an infinite range of active and generally non-toxic medications.

Eclecticism ought truly to be held a virtue in medicine. "One should choose the treatment which seems the best, wherever it may be found" – particularly when it is to be found universally, particularly when such treatment, as in the case with essential oils, commonly possesses a whole variety of properties affecting most often both the part and the whole: the part, because it is their general characteristic that they are able to act on the whole; the whole, because they have dealt successfully with the part. Paul Foulquié put it this way: "An organism is not simply a juxtaposition of tissues. It constitutes a whole and functions as a whole. An organ never acts alone . . . an organism is not a machine whose components each perform their task without reference to the work of the others: in a living being, the parts are involved with the whole . . . a machine is made, while an organism makes itself, and does so over and over again."

Let me assure you that nothing could be further from me than the childish desire to deny to other forms of treatment the great benefits they bring. Quite the reverse: for I am in the market for anything which is able to cure or alleviate without harm.

Nor in any sense would I make the claim that this book is a definitive study of the essential oils. Bearing in mind Trousseau's famous dictum, "Gentlemen, a little more art and a little less science", I have restricted myself to certain essences, since pharmacological research is not yet sufficient to ensure an adequate presentation.

Those I have mentioned have the merit of having been used since time immemorial and of being still in daily use among countless doctors.

As research and experiment continue in the future, their number can only grow. Even at present we nevertheless possess, in aromatherapy, a priceless tool.

This is all the more true since the effect of the essences is not limited to curing or alleviating. By the changes they bring to the body, they act as peerless prophylactic agents against the greatest variety of diseases.

Peerless, and permanent too, if we cultivate the habit of using aromatics daily in the preparation of our food.

It is not my intention to dwell here on what makes good bread; on the desirability of growing vegetables without the anarchic outpouring of pesticides which we see all too often; on the necessity of obtaining pure oils for consumption; nor do I want to discuss what constitutes wholesome food. I shall content myself here with saying, once more, that a well-planned menu should know how to make use of herbs and spices while being aware of the properties of the essences they contain.

Hippocrates taught that it is not enough to anticipate an illness to cure it; one must teach good health to preserve it. Aromatics have always played a leading part in the maintenance of health. And this notion has never been devalued, for, as a Wallachian saying goes, "sickness comes in by a door as wide as a cartwheel and leaves by a crack as narrow as the eye of a needle".

9. Glossary of Main Medical Terms used in this Book.

Abortifacient: capable of inducing an abortion.

Abscess, Cold: slow-forming abscess without accompanying inflammation (tuberculosis, mycosis, i.e. conditions caused by microscopic fungoid growths).

Abscess, Hot: accumulation of pus, with accompanying acute inflammation.

Absorbent: a substance which, internally, combines with gastric secretions and, externally absorbs secretions from wounds (e.g. chalk, carbon).

Adenitis: acute or chronic inflammation of the lymph glands (cervical (neck), inguinal (groin), etc).

Adenoids: enlargement of glandular tissue at the back of the neck.

Adrenal gland: suprarenal gland; one of a pair of endocrine glands situated above each kidney and consisting of two organs, medulla and cortex. The *adrenal cortex* forms numerous hormones which influence the chemical processes in the body, in particular cortisol and aldosterone, known as *corticosteroids.*

Adynamia: extreme muscular weakness accompanying certain diseases.

Aerophagy: swallowing of air.

Agranulocytosis: a condition in which there is a marked decrease or complete disappearance of the white corpuscles of the blood (almost always fatal).

Albuminuria: the presence of alubumin in the urine, occurring e.g. in renal disease and most feverish conditions.

Alcohol: product of the fermentation of vegetable matter containing sugar. Used as a stimulant and vulnerary, etc. Formerly known as "spirits of wine" or "proof spirit".

Alkali (or base): a chemical principle opposed to acids (a base destroys an acid, an acid destroys a base).

Allergy: any noxious modification of body fluids caused by some foreign substance (e.g. medicines, nail varnish, certain foodstuffs).

Alopecia: baldness. There are many causes, for instance: infectious diseases, seborrhoea, tinea, syphilis.

Amaurosis: blindness in which there are no discernible changes in the structure of the eye (caused by albumin, diabetes, anaemia, hysteria, rheumatism, syphilis and alcoholism).

Amenorrhoea: absence of menstruation outside pregnancy in pre-menopausal women. It may be *primary* (when periods have never occurred) or *secondary* (after menses have been established), the menopause excepted.

Amnesia: partial or total loss of memory.

Amoebiasis: parisitic disease caused by the *Entamoeba histolytica.* Local to the large intestine (amoebic dysentery), it may attack other internal organs, e.g. liver, lungs, kidneys, spleen, brain.

Analeptic: medicine or food which restores vitality and stimulates the functioning of the different systems of the body.

Analgesia: the abolition of sensitivity to pain.

Analgesic: a remedy which relieves pain, a pain-killer.

Anaphrodisiac: reducing sexual desire.

Anasarca: dropsy of the cellular tissues which produces general swelling of the body and limbs.

Angina: an inflammation of the throat causing pain on swallowing.

Angina pectoris: syndrome characterised by attacks of severe constricting pains in the region of the chest in front of the heart and radiating down the left arm, accompanied by extreme distress with a feeling of imminent death. Almost always caused by arteriosclerosis of the coronary arteries.

Angina pectoris, False: see Pseudo-angina.

Angiocholitis: inflammation of the bile duct.

Angioma (naevus): small erectile innocent tumour produced by dilation of the capillaries.

Ankylosis: abnormal consolidation and immobility of the bones of a joint.

Ankylostoma duodenale: a small cylindrical worm (hookworm genus), which attaches itself in large numbers to the mucous membrane of the small intestine and causes *ankylostomiasis* (anaemia brought about by numerous and repeated minor haemorrhages), also known as miner's anaemia and hookworm disease.

Anorexia: loss or reduction of appetite.

Anthrax: infectious disease, common to man and animals, caused by a microbe known as the anthrax bacillus (*Bacillus anthracis*). The disease is generally very serious. (Walnut leaves have a bactericidal effect locally on the anthrax pustule).

Antibiotic: literally "hostile to life", the term is used of substances which prevent the development of microbes.

Antibody: the name given to certain substances which appear in animal or human serum following the injection of foreign bodies (microbes, various elements). Some antibodies exist naturally in the serum. These help to defend the organism, their role being principally to bind, dissolve and neutralise microbes or their toxins.

Anthelmintic: destroying or expelling worms; a vermifuge.

Antigen: any substance which stimulates the production of an antibody (q.v.). Microbial germs and any foreign elements in a normal serum may be antigens.

Antipholgisitic: a medication which combats inflammation (medicinal baths, poultices, fomentations, leeches, etc).

Antipruritic: relieving itching.

Antiscorbutic: a remedy or preventive for scurvy.

Antiseptic: that which destroys and prevents the development of microbes.

Antispasmodic: preventing spasms, convulsions, nervous disorders.

Antitussive: relieving coughs.

Aphonia: loss of voice.

Aphrodisiac: substance which arouses sexual desire.

Apoplexy: sudden loss of consciousness and power of movement; temporary or permanent paralysis may result.

Arrhythmia: irregular beating of the heart.

Arteriole: a small artery.

Arteriosclerosis: the thickening and hardening of the arterial walls.

Arteritis: inflammation of an artery.

Arthritis: acute or chronic inflammation of the joints.

Arthritism: that condition of the organism which predisposes it to gout, rheumatism, migraine, asthma, lithiasis, obesity and diabetes.

Ascites: abdominal dropsy; an accumulation of fluid in the peritoneal cavity.

Asthenia, see Debility.

Astringent: agent which causes contraction of organic tissues, reduces secretions and helps formation of scars by preventing inflammation (in cases of haemorrhage, diarrhoea, wounds, leucorrhoea, etc).

Atheroma: sebaceous cyst, small encysted tumour, wen. Also used nowadays to denote degeneration of the arteries: a chronic lesion of the arteries characterised by the formation on the internal walls of yellowish plaques of fatty deposit (cholesterol). These constitute the first stage of arteriosclerosis which often attacks the aorta, the coronary arteries and the arteries of the limbs, and can cause complete closing up. This condition is known as *atherosclerosis.*

Atony: lessening of the normal tone of a contractile organ, e.g. the stomach.

Autonomic nervous systems: consists of the sympathetic and parasympathetic nerves which control involuntary muscles and glandular secretion over which there is no conscious control.

Azotaemia: morbid state in which urea and other nitrogenous waste products are found to excess in the blood.

Azoturia: increase of urea in the urine.

Bactericide: an agent that kills bacteria (one type of microbe).

265

Bacteriostatic: action of the substances which halt the division (reproduction) of bacteria, bringing about their ageing and death.

Balneotherapy: treatment of illnesses by means of medicinal baths (see under Baths, Chapter 7).

Balsamic: fragrant substance imbued with balm and resins, which softens phlegm.

Basedow's disease: exophthalmic goitre; hyperthyroidism with marked protrusion of the eyeballs.

Bile: a secretion of the liver stored in the gall-bladder from which it passes into the intestine, where it aids digestion.

Biliary: Pertaining to bile. *B. ducts:* the tubes through which the bile passes from the liver and gall-bladder to the intestine.

Bilious: a condition caused by excessive secretion of bile, and its regurgitation into the stomach with catarrh of that organ.

Bitters: tonic, aperitif and depurative, prepared from plants. Revitalises the organs (wormwood, centaury, chicory, dandelion, etc).

Blepharitis: inflammation of the eyelids.

Bradycardia: abnormal slowing down of the heartbeat (to less than 60 beats per minute). A condition which be normal or pathological.

Bright's disease: chronic nephritis (multiple dropsy, albuminaria, morbid structural change in the kidneys).

Bulbar: pertaining to the medulla oblongata.

Cachexia: profound alteration of the organism characterised by marked emaciation – "the culmination of all suffering and the outcome of all illness".

Calculus: see Lithiasis.

Calmative: a tranquilliser.

Cancer: a general term to describe malignant growths in tissues, of which *carcinoma* is of epithelial (surface layer of cells either of the skin or of lining tissues), and *sarcoma* of connective tissue origin, as in bone and muscle. A cancerous growth is one which is not encapsulated, but infiltrates into surrounding tissues, the cells of which it replaces by its own.

Carbolic acid: Phenol. An excellent disinfectant (from 2 to 5g to 500g water), used to treat wounds and gangrene, and equally as a household disinfectant, especially for lavatories and drains (long considered the standard disinfectant).

Cardiopathy: any disease of the heart.

Cardiotonic: substance which tones up the heart (cardiac tonic).

Cardiovascular: concerning the heart and blood vessels; of an agent: active in the treatment of diseases of the heart and blood-vessels.

Carminative: agent (aromatic) which causes expulsion of intestinal gas, i.e. relieves flatulence.

Catarrh: inflammation of a mucous membrane accompanied by an excessive discharge of mucus.

Cautery: artificial ulceration on the surface of the skin caused by a caustic agent (counter-irritant). Instrument for burning organic tissue.

Cellulitis: streptococcal inflammation of cellular tissue.

Chancre: the hard swelling that constitutes the primary lesion in syphilis.

Chemotherapy: the specific treatment of disease by the administration of chemical compounds.

Chlorosis: "green sickness"; a type of anaemia found mostly in girls.

Chloraemia: the normal presence of chlorides in the blood; equally, an excess of chlorides in the blood.

Cholaemia: the presence of bile in the blood, causing jaundice.

Cholagogue: agent that aids the evacuation of bile from the biliary ducts and, particularly, the gall-bladder.

Cholecystitits: inflammation of the gall-bladder.

Choleretic: agent which increases secretion of bile.

Cholesterol: a sterol (non-saponifiable fat) found in nervous tissue, red blood corpuscles, animal fat and bile.

Chorea: nervous symptoms characterised by involuntary muscular contractions; St Vitus's dance.

Cicatrising: helping the formation of scar tissue; healing.

Cirrhosis: a degenerative change which can occur in any organ, but especially in the liver; term denoting hepatic disorders of various origins (e.g. alcoholic cirrhosis, tubercular cirrhosis, malarial cirrhosis, etc).

Colic: severe pain due to spasmodic contraction of the involuntary muscle of tubes, e.g. intestinal colic.

Colitis: a condition of inflammation of the colon.

Compress: folded material, e.g. lint, wet or dry, applied to a part of the body.

Condyloma: small cutaneous tumour occuring in the region of the anus or genital organs.

Congestion: an accumulation of blood in any part of the body.

Contagious disease: disease spread from one person to another by direct contact.

Contusion: a bruise, injury to deeper tissues through intact skin.

Cordial: a stimulant and tonic (all aromatic plants are cordial).

A formula for medicinal cordial:

red wine	125g
tincture of cinnamon	8g
simple syrup	25g

Coronaritis: inflammation of the coronary arteries, causing a predisposition to *Angina pectoris.*

Cortex: the external layer of an organ.

Coryza: cold in the head, with headache, nasal catarrh, and purulent discharge.

Counter-irritant: medication or treatment whose purpose is to draw to one part of the body fluids which are blocking another part (leeches, vesicants, mustard plasters, cupping, purgatives); irritant used to relieve another irritation.

Cutaneous: pertaining to the skin.

Cystitis: inflammation of the bladder.

Cytophylactic: (*cyto-* as a prefix denoting or relating to the cells) substances which protect the cells of an organism. (Magnesium and the aromatic essences are cytophylactics.)

Debility: a condition of feebleness, weakness and lack of physical tone; general state of depression entailing multiple functional deficiencies.

Depurative: substance which combats impurity of the blood and the internal organs (diuretics, sudorifics).

Dermatosis: any skin disease.

Detersive: detergent; that which cleanses wounds, sores and ulcers, promoting the formation of scar tissue.

Diaphoretic: see Sudorific.

Diathesis: constitutional predisposition to certain diseases (e.g. arthritic or tubercular diathesis). Synonymous with Temperament.

Digestive: digestive stimulant. Substance which stimulates digestion (most aromatics are stimulants).

Diuresis: discharge of urine. (Also, excessive discharge of urine.)

Diuretic: substance which aids production of urine.

Drastic: a violent purgative.

Dropsy: excess of fluid in the tissues or in a natural cavity of the body (abdomen, meninges). Hydropsy. See also *Ascites, Oedema.*

Dyscrasia: constitutional weakness. *Blood d.*, a developmental disorder of the blood.

Dyshidrosis: skin disease local to the area between the fingers, characterised by a recurrent vesicular rash and caused by a disturbance of the sweat mechanism.

Dysmenorrhoea: painful and difficult menstruation.

Dyspepsia: painful and difficult digestion.

Dyspnoea: difficulty in breathing.

Dystonia: condition affecting tonicity or tonus (e.g. dystonia of the sympathetic nervous system).

Ecchymosis: an effusion of blood in the tissues, generally as a result of contusion; bruising.

Emetic: an agent which has power to induce vomiting.

Emmenagogue: substance which induces or regularises menstruation.

Emollient: a substance which softens the tissue, soothes inflammation and refreshes the areas with which it is in contact.

Emphysema: the abnormal presence of air in tissues or cavities of the body. *Pulmonary emphysema:* a chronic disease of the lungs in which there is abnormal distension of the alveoli; an accompaniment of chronic respiratory diseases, in which narrowing of the tubes occurs.

Endocarditis: inflammation of the endocardium (the membrane lining the heart).

Engorgement: congestion.

Enteritis: inflammation of the intestine.

Enuresis: incontinence of urine, almost always during sleep (nocturnal).

Epigastrium: that region of the abdomen which is situated over the stomach.

Epistaxis: bleeding from the nose.

Erythema: skin congestion.

Erethism: abnormal irritability.

Eupeptic: substance which aids digestion.

Exutory: artificial ulcer maintained as a counter-irritant in an illness.

Febrifuge: agent which combats fever and staves off its return.

Fistula, Anal: an abnormal passage resulting from an abscess, connecting the anus to the skin.

Flatulence: abundance of gas in the stomach and intestine accompanied by swelling.

Furunculosis: a staphylococcal infection represented by many, or crops of, boils.

Galactagogue: medicament or foodstuff which promotes secretion of milk.

Gangrene: death of tissue.

Gastralgia: stomach pain of neuralgic type.

Gastritis: inflammation of the mucous membrane lining the stomach.

Genito-urinary: referring to both the reproductive organs and the urinary tract.

Glossitis: acute or chronic inflammation of the tongue.

Gout: a metabolic disease associated with an excess of uric acid in the blood.

Gravel: renal concretions, normally the size of a pin-head. Smaller concretions form *sand*; those which are larger become *calculi* (stones).

Haematemesis: vomiting of blood from the stomach.

Haematoma: an effusion of blood enclosed in a cyst.

Haematuria: passing of blood in the urine.

Haemolytic: that which destroys the red blood corpuscles.

Haemophilia: hereditary disease transmitted by women and affecting only men, characterised by a disposition to prolonged haemorrhage from the least injury.

Haemopoiesis: the formation of red blood cells.

Haemoptysis: vomiting of blood of pulmonary origin.

Haemorrhage: an escape of blood from its vessels.

Haemorrhoids: piles; locally dilated rectal veins.

Haemostatic: that which arrests bleeding.

Health (F. Hoffman's precepts for good health):
    1 – avoid all excess.
    2 – avoid sudden change of habit.
    3 – keep a calm light-hearted spirit (the best guarantee).
    4 – seek out pure air and a temperate climate (for body and mind).
    5 – know what food to eat.
    6 – work out a balance between food and physical exercise.
    7 – shun excessive recourse to medicines and doctors.

269

Hepatic: relating to the liver.

Hepatitis: inflammation of the liver common in tropical countries (Amoebic hepatitis).

Hippocras: stimulant drink with a base of sugared wine and aromatic plants.

Humoral: pertaining to a bodily fluid or *humour.*

Hydrotherapy: treatment of disease by water in all its forms and at various temperatures. Indicated in numerous conditions, e.g. anaemia, general fatigue, gout, hysteria, obesity.

Given in the form of baths, douches, steam baths, frictions, affusions, etc.

Affusions: with the temperature of the water at 10–12°C, start with a period of 15 seconds and increase gradually without exceeding one minute. Follow with friction rubbing all over and 20 minutes of exercises to bring about the reaction.

Apart from its therapeutic properties, hydrotherapy is a preventive of colds, neuralgia and pulmonary diseases.

Hypertension: raised blood pressure.

Hypertensive: agent which raises blood pressure.

Hypnotic: agent which causes sleep.

Hypochondria: morbid preoccupation with one's health; also, general debility whose cause is related to a disorder of the organs situated in the hypochondrium (the upper region of the abdomen on each side of the epigastrium), e.g. liver, stomach.

Hypotension: low blood pressure.

Hypotensive: agent which lowers blood pressure.

Hypoglycaemia: less than normal blood-sugar.

Infarct: term applied to a vascular region where circulation has become blocked (e.g. pulmonary infarct, intestinal infarct). *Myocardial infarct, infarction*; intra-myocardial haemorrhage caused by closure of one branch of the coronary artery.

Intercostal: between the ribs. *Intercostal muscles:* those of the chest wall.

Intermittent fever: fever which recurs at greater or lesser intervals (chiefly malaria, but sometimes also suppurating hepatitis, urinary infection, purulent infection); the term is often used as a synonym for malaria.

Keratitis: inflammation of the cornea.

Koch's bacillus: the *Mycobacterium tuberculosis*, causative organism of tuberculosis.

Lard (as used in formulae): purified pig-fat (an ingredient of ointments, unguents, etc).

Lactation: the process of milk secretion.

Lacteal: of milk.

Lavage: washing out a cavity.

Lesion: an injury, wound or morbid structural change in an organ. The word is used as a general term for some local disease condition.

Leucocyte: a white blood corpuscle.

Leucocytosis: increased number of leucocytes in the blood.

Leucoma: a white spot on the cornea, following an injury to the eye.

Leucorrhoea: a thick whitish discharge from the vagina, "the whites".

Lithiasis: condition which involves the formation of sand or small stones in a gland or reservoir (renal, i.e. kidney or urinary, lithiasis; salivary lithiasis; biliary lithiasis, etc).

Lymphatism: of sluggish and flabby disposition, once supposed to result from excess of lymph.

Macerate: to steep or soak, to soften by steeping.

Medulla oblongata: that portion of the spinal cord which is contained inside the cranium (part of the skull). In it are the nerve centres which govern respiration and the action of the heart, etc.

Membrane: a thin elastic tissue covering the surface of certain organs and lining the cavities of the body.

Meninges: the membranes covering the brain and spinal cord.

Menopause: the change of life, the cessation of the menstrual function.

Menorrhagia: excessive periods.

Menstrual cycle: oestrous cycle in women; periodic modification of the uterus and vagina, triggered by ovarian secretions which prepare for fertilisation and pregnancy.

Meteorism: distension of the abdomen by intestinal gas.

Metritis: inflammation of the uterus.

Metrorrhagia: uterine haemorrhage occuring outside menstrual periods.

Microbe: a minute living organism, especially those causing disease: bacteria, viruses, etc.

Micturition: the action of urinating.

Mycosis: any parasitic disease caused by a fungus.

Myocarditis: inflammation of myocardium (muscle tissue of the heart).

Narcotic: that which induces sleep and eases suffering (poisonous in high doses). Synonyms: stupefacient, soporific.

Nephritis: acute or chronic inflammation of the kidneys.

Neuralgia: sharp stabbing pain along the course of a nerve, owing to neuritis or functional disturbance.

Neurasthenia: nervous exhaustion; general (physical and mental) debility.

Neuritis: inflammation of a nerve.

Nymphomania: exaggerated sexual desire in a woman.

Odontalgia: toothache.

Oedema: serous infiltration of the tissues. In the region of the skin it is characterised by painless swelling.

Oestrogen: hormone responsible for the oestrous cycle in women (menstrual cycle) and female mammals.

Officinal: used in medicine; recognised in the pharmacopoeia.

Oliguria: diminution in the amount of urine secreted.

Ophthalmia: inflammation of the eye, characterised by redness.

271

Ophthalmic: relating to the eye.

Otitis: inflammation of the ear.

Otorrhoea: discharge from the ear.

Palpitation: rapid and forceful contraction of the heart.

Panacea: a cure-all.

Parasympathetic system: part of the autonomic nervous system (q.v.).

Paresis: partial paralysis.

Pectoral: relating to the chest; of a treatment, beneficial to the respiratory system.

Peri-anal: surrounding or located around the anus.

Pericarditis: inflammation of the pericardium (the membranous sac enveloping the heart). May be acute or chronic, dry or serous.

Perineal: relating to the perineum, i.e. the tissues between the anus and external genitals.

Peristalsis: contraction which causes the contents of the alimentary canal to move onwards.

Petri dishes: shallow glass dishes in which organisms are grown on a culture medium.

Pharmacopoeia: an authoritative publication which gives the standard formulae and preparation of drugs as used in a given country. *Codex.*

Phlebitis: inflammation of a vein which tends to formation of a thrombus.

Phthisis: pulmonary tuberculosis.

Phytotherapy: the treatment of disease by plants; herbal therapy.

Plethora: excess of blood or humours throughout the whole body or in one part.

Pneumonia: inflammation of the lung.

Pneumothorax: air in the pleural cavity causing collapse of the lung.

Potassium bromide: chemical substance of great value in the treatment of epilepsy, spermatorrhoea, nervousness, St Vitus's dance, morning sickness et al. (2 to 4g).

Prophylactic: preventive of disease.

Prostatitis: inflammation of the prostate gland (the gland surrounding the male urethra at its juction with the bladder and associated with the genital organs).

Prurigo: chronic skin disease with an irritating papular eruption.

Pruritis: itching.

Pseudo-angina: false angina pectoris; pain experienced in the region over the heart by anxious individuals without evidence of organic heart disease.

Psoriasis: a chronic skin disease characterised by reddish patches with profuse silvery scaling, chiefly on knees and elbows.

Psychasthenia: mental disorder, characterised by indecisiveness, tendency to doubt and to irrational fears, which leads to various phobias.

Psychosomatic (medicine): the study of mental disturbance of emotional type and of the visceral disorders which are its physical manifestations.

Puerperal: relating to childbirth.

Pulmonary: pertaining to or affecting the lungs.

Purgative: substance which produces evacuation of the bowels.

Purulent: forming, containing or resembling pus.

Pyelonephritis: inflammation of the renal pelvis and kidney.

Renal: relating to the kidney.

Resolvent: agent which disperses swelling (iodides, aromatic plants, alcohol).

Revulsive: see Counter-irritant.

Rhinitis: inflammation of the mucous membrane of the nose.

Rubefacient: an agent causing redness of the skin.

Salpingitis: acute or chronic inflammation of the Fallopian tubes.

Sarcoma: see Cancer.

Scab: a dark crust formed of dead tissue, which is self-eliminating.

Sclerosis: the hardening of any part from an overgrowth of fibrous and connective tissues.

Scrofula: tuberculosis, especially of the lymphatic glands ("King's evil").

Scrofulosis: a type of lymphatic temperament peculiar to childhood and adolescence characterised by a predisposition to common skin diseases (impetigo) and mucous infections (rhinitis, otitis, etc), sweating and a chronic aspect, and equally a predisposition to tuberculosis localised in the ganglia, bones and joints and evolving with slight reaction.

Seborrhoea: increased secretion of the sebaceous glands (encouraging acne, baldness, etc).

Sedative: agent which lessens excitement or functional activity.

Senescence: the process of growing old.

Spermatorrhoea: involuntary emission of sperm.

Starch: extracted from corn, rice or maize, it is absorbent and used in poultices, washes and medicinal baths.

Sternutatory: agent which provokes sneezing and the secretion of nasal mucus (nasal sympathetic therapy).

Stomachic: digestive aid; gastric tonic.

Stomatitis: inflammation of the mucous membrane of the mouth (redness, salivation, ulceration).

Secondary infection: a new infection contracted by a subject already infected and not yet cured.

Sudorific: an agent causing sweating.

Sympathetic nervous system: a branch of the autonomic nervous system which supplies involuntary muscle and glands.

Synergy: the harmonious action of two agents working together.

Tachycardia: accelerated rhythm of the heartbeat.

Taenia: tapeworm.

Thrombosis: the formation of a thrombus.

Thrombus: a stationary blood-clot caused by coagulation of the blood, usually in a vein.

273

Thrush: aphthae; an infection of the mucous membrane of the mouth by a fungus and characterised by small white superficial ulcers.

Tracheitis: inflammation of the windpipe.

Urticaria: nettle-rash or hives.

Vagus: the tenth cranial nerve arising in the medulla and providing the para-sympathetic nerve supply to the organs in the thorax and abdomen.

Valetudinarian: person of a delicate constitution.

Vasoconstrictor: that which contracts the blood vessels.

Vasodilator: agent which causes increase in the lumen (calibre) of blood vessels.

Vegetation: a plant-like growth. *Adenoid vegetation:* overgrowth of lymphoid tissue in the nasopharynx.

Vermifuge: an agent which expels intestinal worms.

Vesicant: vesicatory; a blistering plaster applied to the skin to provoke a counter-irritant serosity.

Vesicle: a blister or small sac usually containing fluid.

Virus, Filtrable: microbial germ so small that it passes through the filters normally used to study microbes and is not visible under a microscope. Poliomyelitis, aphthous fever, shingles and chicken-pox are caused by filtrable viruses.

Vulnerary: an agent which heals wounds and sores by external administration.

White tumour: white swelling; chronic tubercular arthritis.

Appendices

1. Embalming in the Age of the Pharoahs

While he was in Egypt, Herodotus studied the medicine of the priests and the practice of embalming, and gave a detailed account.

There were, he found, many accredited embalmers. "When a body is brought to them, they produce specimen models in wood painted to resemble nature." The most sought-after represented Osiris; these were the most expensive. Other models of all sorts were shown, down to the cheapest.

He then describes the embalming techniques. First the brain was extracted through the nostrils with an iron hook; what could not be extracted was rinsed out with appropriate drugs inserted into the head. "Next the flank is laid open with a flint knife and the whole contents of the abdomen removed; the cavity is then thoroughly cleansed and washed out, first with palm wine and again with an infusion of pounded spices. After that it is filled with pure bruised myrrh, cinnamon, and every other aromatic substance with the exception of frankincense, and sewn up again, after which the body is placed in natrum, covered entirely over, for seventy days – never longer." Then the body was washed and wrapped in strips of linen smeared on the underside with gum, and given back to the family in a wooden case shaped like the human figure to be placed upright in a sepulchral chamber. This, according to Herodotus, was the first-class or superior method of embalming.

For less wealthy families, oil of cedar was injected into the stomach of the corpse, without the removal of the contents. The body was then pickled for seventy days, after which the oil was extracted and the corpse returned to the relatives.

Herodotus adds that the Egyptians believed that corpses so prepared would be preserved for longer than the prophetic 3,000 years – the term fixed for a soul's escape from metempsychosis. The corpses of the mummies in the Louvre and elsewhere prove the Egyptians accurate in their calculations.

2. Aspirin Reactions

All substances, even natural ones, are capable of provoking a reaction. I have mentioned a case of urticaria resulting from a few minutes spent under a blossoming lime-tree. Insomnia brought about by drinking an infusion of lime-flowers has also been recorded.

Aspirin cannot be exempted from a list of such substances; indeed, it can cause more serious consequences. I have already cited some examples and have known many cases from my own experience, one of the more recent of which dates from June 1973. Mr M had to be rushed to hospital for the second time in 15 years after ingesting *one single aspirin tablet*, suffering from oedema of the glottis (swollen throat). Death was narrowly avoided.

In 1973 during a "Hospital Week", one of the subjects offered for consideration was "aspirin as an enemy of the stomach". Truly this had been known for a long enough time. It was generally agreed that aspirin must be prescribed and taken with great caution. In a sample taken by Professor Kiepping, 51% of digestive haemorrhages were found to be caused by aspirin – a sizeable figure when compared with those for other anti-inflammatory products (e.g. phenylbutazone, cortisone and derivatives). These latter, incidentally, are far from being exempt from involvement in a variety of complications themselves, some quite serious. To read the scientific accounts over 15 years is enough – the period would have been longer if the author had not been earlier overwhelmed by the bewildering publicity put out by the manufacturers of these products.

The aspirin is universally known; but it would be much better if it were not universally used – as lightly as marsh-mallow or chewing gum. Beware of the deadly habit of swallowing aspirin at the slightest incentive, even though it carries a household name. It has won that household name through advertising: thus is public opinion, ignorant of expert knowledge, formed. If you must take a proprietary medicament, look beneath the brand name and discover its proper scientific name.

Those press resumés should not obscure the justified reputation of the aspirin. They remind us simply that, as Georges Duhamel put it, "*all treatment is experiment*" – and it pays to remember this.

3. Cumin

Cumin (Cuminum cyminum) of the Umbelliferae family, is not an essence prescribed by doctors, but it may be used – and indeed has been for centuries – in cooking.

The dried seeds are used to spice cheese, sausage, bread and pickled cabbage, sometimes in conjunction with juniper berries and fennel.

There is no doubt that cumin is a *digestive stimulant*; it is frequently taken with Munster cheese. It is also antiseptic, antispasmodic and carminative.

Bibliography

This bibliography is necessarily incomplete, for it is not possible to have read every work dealing with plants and aromatic essences. Further, there may be unwitting omissions; if so I apologise to any living author so treated.

Arend G. – Volkstümliche Anwendung der einheimischen Arzneipflanzen. Verlag von Stringer, Berlin, 1925.

Bayle – Formulaire général. "Encyclopédie des Sciences Médicales", Paul Mellier éditeur, 1844.

Benezet L. – Contribution à l'étude de l'essence de lavande, Parfumerie, 1943, I, 153–157.

Binet L. – Au bord de l'étang. Magnard Editeur, Rouen, 1948.

Binet L. – Leçons de Biologie dans un parc. Magnard éditeur, Paris, 1960.

Binet L. – Diététique et gastronomie. Figaro Littéraire, 1963.

Binet L., Bour H. et Tanret P. – Effets comparés des cures de chou et de citron dans le traitement de l'ascite cirrhotique. B. et M. de la Soc. Méd. des Hôpitaux de Paris, 1948, n° 9. – II.

Cadéac C. et Meunier A. – Travaux divers. C. R. Soc. Biol., 1889 à 1892.

Capo N. – Mis observaciones clinicas sobre el limon. Sanch., Barcelona.

Carles P. – Un dernier mot sur l'action diurétique de l'oignon. Gaz. Hebd. des Sc. Méd. de Bordeaux, 1912.

Caujolle – Toulouse Médical, 1943, 44, 483. Annales Pharm, françaises, 1944, 2, 147.

Cavel L. – Sur la valeur antiseptique de quelques huiles essentielles. C R. Acad. Sc., 1918.

Cazal R. – Contribution à l'étude de l'activité pharmacodynamique c quelques essences de labiées. Thèse Toulouse, 1944.

Clarus J. – Handbuch der Speziellen Arzneimittellehre, 1860, Leipzig.

Colin Clair et Maronne M. – Dictionaire des herbes et des épices. Denoël éditeur, Paris, 1963.

Costet P. – Phytothérapie des affections artério-veineuses en pratique phlébologique. Maloine éditeur, Paris, 1963.

Coupin H. – Les plantes médicinales. Costes A. éditeur, Paris, 1920.

Courmont P., Morel A. et Bay I. – Sur le pouvoir infertilisant de quelques essences végétales vis-à-vis du bacille tuberculeux humain. C. R. Soc. Biol., 1927.

Courmont P., Morel A., Perrot L. et Sanlaville S. – Du pouvoir infertilisant de l'essence d'ail et de moutarde sur les cultures homogènes de bacille de Koch. C. R. Soc. Biol., 1937.

Couvreur A. – Les produits aromatiques utilisés en pharmacie. Vigot frères éditeurs, Paris, 1939.

Czapek – Biochimie der Pflanzen, Verlag von Fischer, Iéna, 1922–1923.

Delange R. – Essences nouvelles et parfums. A. Colin, édit., 1930.

Dorvault – L'Officine. Vigot éditeur, Paris, 1945.

Dragendorff G. – Die Heilpflanzen, Verlag Enke, Stuttgart, 1898.

Forgues E. – L'essence déterpénée de lavande contre les plaies anfractueuses. Parfumerie Moderne, 1917.

Fournier P. – Le livre des plantes médicinales et vénéneuses de France. Paul Lechevalier éditeur, Paris, 1948.

Fröhnere – Lerbuch der Arzneimittellehre für Tierärzte. Verlag Enke, Stuttgart, 1911.

Gattefosse R. M. – Antiseptiques essentiels. Girardot éditeur, Paris, 1926.

Gattefosse R. M. – Aromathérapie. Girardot éditeur, Paris, 1928.

Gilberta et Michel Ch. – Formulaire pratique de thérapeutique et de pharmacologie. Doin éditeur, Paris, 1925.

Giral F. et Rojahnc – Productos Quimicos y Farmaceuticos. Editorial Atlante Mexico, 1946.

Goris A., Liot A. et Goris A. – Pharmacie galénique, Masson et Cie éditeurs, Paris, 1942.

Hussmann et Hilgter – Die Pflanzenstoffe. I. Springer, Berlin, 1882.

Jacques R. – Traitement de la tuberculose pulmonaire par la méthode des essences. Marseille Médicale, 1927.

King's – American Dispensatory, 18e édition. The Ohio Valley Company Cincinnati, 317, Race Street, 1898.

Leclerc H. – Les épices. Masson et Cie éditeurs, 1929.

Leclerc H. – Précis de Phytothérapie. Masson éditeur, Paris, 1954.

Lemery – Dictionnaire des drogues simples. 1798.

Martindale et Westcott – The Extra Pharmacopoeia. Lavis and Co, Ltd., London.

Moiroux Jean – Les huiles essentielles en dermatologie vétérinaire. Thèse Lyon, 1943.

Morel A. et Rochaix A. – Nombreuses communications dans Bulletin Sc. Pharmacol. et C. R. Soc. Biol., de 1922 à 1928.

Oesterle – Grundriss der Pharmakochemie. Verlag Bornträger, Berlin, 1909.

Oesterlen F. – Handbuch der Heilmittellehre. Tübingen, 1853.

Perrot Em. – Matières premières du règne végétal. Masson et Cie éditeurs, Paris, 1944.

Mme Porcher-Pimpard – Contribution à l'étude du pouvoir antiseptique des essences végétales. Thèse Toulouse, 1942.

Reynier P. – Travaux divers, 1943.

Rolet A. – Plantes à parfums et plantes aromatiques. J. B. Baillière et fils, édit., 1930.

Schmiedeberg O. – Grundriss der Pharmacologie. Verlag Vogel, Leipzig, 1913.

Schuchart D. B. – Handbuch der Arzneimittellehre und Rezeptierkunt. Vieweg und sohn, Bruaschweig, 1858.

Trendelenburg P. – Grundlagen der Allgem. und Speziellen Arnei-verordnung. Verlag Vogel, Leipzig, 1926.

Trier – Chemie der Pflanzenstoffe. Verlag Bornträger, Berlin, 1924.

Tschirch A. – Handbuch der Pharmakognosie. Verlag Tauchnitz, Leipzig, 1917.

Uebèle G. – Handlexikon der Tierräztlichen Praxis. Verlag Ebner, Ulm, 1921.

Valnet J.:
   – *Traitements des maladies par les légumes, les fruits et les céréales,* 4e édition, Maloine édit., Paris (1973).
   – *Docteur nature,* Fayard édit., Paris (1971).
   – *Phytothérapie,* Maloine édit. 1972.
      et pour mémoire:
   – Le citral-uréthane en dermatologie. L'Essor médico-social dans l'Union Française, juillet 1954.
   – Lithiases et thérapeutique aromatique. L'Hôpital, mai 1959.
   – Cholestérol et thérapeutique aromatique. A.M.I.F., janvier 1960.
   – Phytothérapie et aromathérapie. Leur place dans la thérapeutique actuelle. Les Actualités Médico-Chirurgicales, L'Hôpital, mars 1961.
   – La mésenchymothérapie – L'Hôpital, avril 1961
   – L'aromathérapie et les thérapeutiques naturelles face à la maladie (indications et résultats). L'Hôpital, janvier-mars 1962.

Valnet J. et Reddet Cl. – Contribution à l'application pratique d'une nouvelle conception du terrain biologique. A.M.I.F., avril et mai 1961.

Valnet J., Girault M., Lapraz J.-Cl., Belaiche P., Duraffourd Ch. Phyto-thérapie et aromathérapie."Phytothérapie et Plantes Médicinales", Juin 1973.

Vander – Medicina natural. Sanch. édit., Barcelona.

Waldenburg et Simon – Handbuch der Arzneiverordnungslehre. Verlag Hirschwald, Berlin, 1887.

Wattiez N. et Sternon F. – Eléments de chimie végétale, Masson et Cie édit., Paris, 1935.

Wiesner J. – Rohstoffe der Pflanzenreiches. Verlag Engelmann, Leipzig, 1927.

Wolffenstein – Die Pflanzenalkaloide. Verlag Springer, Berlin, 1922.

Where to Obtain Essential Oils

A comprehensive range of pure essences for aromatherapy is obtainable by direct mail from

Aromatic Oil Company, 12 Littlegate Street, Oxford, England.

For more information on Essential Oils,
Aromatherapy Books, and the complete Aveda
Aromatherapy/Ayurvedic Product Line, contact
the Aveda Corporation.

Aveda Corporation
321 Lincoln Street NE
Minneapolis, MN 55413
(612)379-8500   (800)328-0849

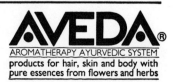

For more information on Essential Oils,
Aromatherapy Book... and the complete Aveda
Aromatherapy/Ayurveda 2001 or The contact
the Aveda Corporation.

Aveda Corporation
4221 Lincoln Street NE
Minneapolis, MN 55111
(612) 270-6300   (800) 3XX-00X0